Looking Great, Staying Young

Looking Great, Staying Young

by
Dick Clark

with Bill Libby

The Bobbs-Merrill Company, Inc.

Indianapolis/New York

Library of Congress Cataloging in Publication Data

Clark, Dick, 1929-
    Looking great, staying young.

    1. Middle aged men — Health and hygiene. 2.
Grooming for men. I. Title.
RA777.8.C57   613'.04234   80-684
ISBN 0-672-52657-3

        Designed by Jacques Chazaud
    Manufactured in the United States of America

            First Printing

For my parents,
whom I selected very carefully!

Acknowledgments

The authors wish to thank Dick's wife, Kari Clark; Dick's secretary, Priscilla Abeyte; the transcriber, Jackie Sommers; Drs. William Klein, Lloyd Singer, and William Harrison; Bruce Geller, Marge Swenson, Lucy Kohn, Kenneth Craig, Jean Donielle, and Arthur Ellen; and all others who contributed to this book, including Grace Shaw and Irene Glynn, who edited it.

Contents

Looking Great, Staying Young

1

Staying Young

I'm fifty-one and I look thirty. At least that's what people say, and it's what I see when I look in the mirror. At fifty, I still feel like I did when I was thirty. I was born November 30, 1929, and I consider myself lucky to look and feel twenty years younger than I am.

Although I've done and am doing many other things, I'm known primarily as host of television's "American Bandstand." Originally, it was a local show in Philadelphia. It started in 1952, almost thirty years ago. It's been on nationally since the summer of 1957.

It's one of the oldest and longest-

running shows on network television,
and I've been doing it since I was
twenty-seven. But people are always telling me I don't look any older than when
they watched me in the early days, and
they ask me what the secrets of this success are.

I've had people who used to watch
the show in the old days ask me if I was
Dick Clark's son carrying on for good old
dad. And I've had little old ladies and
gray-haired gents tell me they've been
watching me for twenty-some years, and
a few have asked me how come I look so
good when I have to be so old. One man
said, "I'm over the hill, so you must be.
But you don't look it." I have to admit I'm
happy to hear it.

The other day I was signing autographs after a fairgrounds show when a
lad of about high school age asked me if I
remembered so-and-so. When I said I
didn't, he said they were his parents and
they used to dance on my show once in
a while. They weren't regulars or I'd
probably have remembered them, but
the grown-up children of people who
used to watch my show or were on my
show keep popping up. I feel like a high
school teacher who's starting to see a
second generation of his students turn
up in his classes.

I don't feel old. I guess I'm getting
there, but I'm going to go as slowly as
possible. A lot of feeling young and look-

ing young is in the mind. They say you're as old as you feel.

Recently I was reminiscing with an audience about the early years of the show when a little boy, who looked too young to stand, stood up and said, "Mr. Clark, I've been watching you for years." We all laughed because the kid looked like his oldest memory couldn't go back past Thursday, but I guess the little guy was old for his size.

When I get into an audience participation portion of a show, people often do ask how come I've aged so little. I say, "I owe it all to clean living." It's always good for a laugh. When I get right to it, however, I admit I picked my parents very carefully. I've been blessed with the good luck of having come from good bloodlines.

My mom was a young-looking lady who was active until she died of a heart attack in her middle seventies. My dad is a young-looking guy who is still going strong in his middle eighties.

I'm no Paul Newman, but, to be honest, I don't think I'm Alfred E. Newman, either. And, frankly, I think a lot of looking good, looking young is the luck of the draw. I got good genes from my parents. I guess I have good body chemistry.

I keep a hectic schedule. I host "American Bandstand" every Saturday afternoon, and hosted the "$20,000 Pyramid" every weekday afternoon for a

long time. I have my own production
company, which does a lot of TV specials
and theater movies. And we package live
shows for coast-to-coast tours.

I have offices in Hollywood and in
New York City and travel coast to coast
every week or two, and I tour cross-
country from time to time. I don't seem
to tire out. I seem to have endless energy.

A lot of people look young on the
outside but are old inside. Others look
old on the outside but are young inside. I
haven't had any health problems. I guess
I'm one of the lucky ones, inside and
outside.

I'm not the only lucky one, of course.
A lot of television and movie stars maintain their youthful looks. People talk
about Pat Boone like they talk about me.
But, as I tell Pat, he's just a kid! Pat's only
forty-six.

Michael Landon is forty-three, Ryan
O'Neal and Larry Hagman are forty-nine,
Robert Wagner is fifty, and James Garner
is fifty-two.

Alan Alda is forty-five, Johnny Carson
is fifty-four, Paul Newman is fifty-six,
Monty Hall is fifty-eight, and Charles
Bronson and Tony Randall are sixty-one.

Looking young is true of a lot of
ladies, too. Valerie Harper is forty, Ann
Margret is forty-one, Mary Tyler Moore
is forty-three and Angie Dickinson is
forty-four. Dinah Shore, who looks super,
is sixty-three.

As I suggested, a lot of looking and staying young is luck and heredity. But I have seen what some performers do to stay young in a profession that demands a good appearance, and there are things I do that help me maintain my youthful looks and attitude. There are some secrets I can reveal to you that may help you.

I've been asked about how I stay young-looking so much, I decided to do a book about it. This is it.

I don't pretend to be an expert, but I have asked some experts to contribute. I have thought about youthful looks and a youthful attitude a lot and have come to some conclusions about it.

There's a lot to it. It's not just the looks you were born with, of course. Or the chemistry to keep these healthy.

There's a lot we can do to keep ourselves in shape. There's vigorous exercise and a good diet. Frankly, I'm not a physical fitness nut. I like to eat, and I don't like to sweat. But few people have to be fat. Most of us can get trim if we want it enough. It may seem strange to you, but I fast frequently. It allows me to cheat at times.

You can get good medical and dental care. I do.

How good are vitamins for you? How bad are drugs? I've looked into it. I don't smoke anymore, although I did for years. I drink a little. I used to drink a lot. I'll get into this later in this book.

5

You can take care of your teeth and your hair and your skin. You can brush your teeth, and brush your hair, and cleanse your skin. I use face cream, like the ladies. Why shouldn't a man? I get my hair styled at a beauty parlor. Why not? I buy good clothes and get them fit to me.

There even are extreme things you can do to make yourselves look better. If you have bad teeth, have them straightened or capped or replaced. If your hair isn't as you want it, change the color of it or wear a wig or a hairpiece. I went to the experts to give you practical advice in this book on everything from fashions to plastic surgery. If you think it would improve your appearance, get a nose-bob or an ear-trim or a face-lift. Why not? I'm not unhappy with my nose or my ears, but if I were, I'd get them fixed. I haven't had a face-lift because I haven't needed it. If I do, I will. And I won't be one bit embarrassed about it. If a woman wants to enlarge or reduce her breasts, get a tummy-tuck, or things like that, I think she should.

This book is aimed primarily at men, but much of the advice will apply to women as well. As a man, I keep a keen eye on women. For whatever it's worth, I know what I like in a lady. I have watched and worked with and been friendly with some of the most youthful-looking ladies in show business. I have asked them about the things they do to look so great, and here and there I will throw in some words of wisdom to any women who may be in the audience.

If you're not happy with yourself as you are, and there are things that you can do to improve yourself, why not do them? I think it's important to be as happy with yourself as possible. I think it's reflected in the way you look and feel.

I know some things you can do and I've looked into other things to find out how hard they are to do, how much they will cost, and how predictable the results are. I'll pass on to you what I found out.

I'm not saying you can stop the clock, but I believe you can turn it back a bit. I'm not going to tell you that you can look like a television star, but I really believe that most people can look better than they do. I'll bet *you* can.

A lot of looking good lies in how you package the product. A man doesn't have to be young to dress like a young man.

But, you don't have to overdo it.

A young man in his twenties or thirties doesn't have to wear a dark, drab business suit simply because he's in business. He can look like he's serious and also wear suits in the current cuts and colors.

And a fellow in his forties can keep up with fashions without trying to look like a teen-ager. It is important to keep up with the fashions.

No one looks more foolish than a fellow in his fifties standing by the barbecue in plaid shorts, long socks and shiny shoes. Or wearing gold chains and a shirt open to his navel with the white hairs on his chest showing. There are things he can wear that are youthful, lively, and also stylish, and we'll get into those in this book.

You may not look like Clark Gable or Rock Hudson, but you can look younger and better than you now do, and you'll feel better and younger. A lot about age is in the mind, and I believe you have to work at thinking younger.

I think you have to talk to young people to know what they are thinking. What's more important, you have to listen to them. I do, but I don't think most people do.

My show keeps me in contact with teen-agers. Times change, and so do teen-agers. If I didn't listen to them, my show wouldn't change with them and would die. So, it comes naturally to me, and I advise you to follow my lead.

I also deal with singers and dancers and actors and directors and producers and advertising people and business people of all ages. I listen to them and learn from them. So, too, you can listen to the experts of your world.

I read a great deal, too. And I try to keep up with the trends so that I can deal with people of all ages in all the professions on equal terms.

I don't look down on a guy or gal in his or her twenties because I've learned there are prodigies in every profession. I don't look up to every veteran of sixty or seventy because I know that some of them *think* old.

I have never stopped doing the things I like to do. I think too many people do. They stop going to movies, the theater, concerts, and such because they think they've seen it all. But there are always shows and stars to see that are new and different.

I'm in a line of work with unlimited horizons. I can try to do not only better shows, but different kinds of shows. No matter what you work at, you can try to do different things that may be better and may give you the chance to do better work.

It's too easy to sink into ruts. People stop taking vacations because "they've been there." But there have to be places they *haven't* been. There have to be experiences they *haven't* had. You don't have to try everything, but there are bound to be new things to try that will be interesting to you.

Because you've had sex, are you going to give it up? I've had my share, but I haven't had enough. The only thing I've had enough of is wives. I've been married three times. I'm not proud of it. But because two marriages didn't work didn't mean I wasn't going to try another.

I've lived with women I wasn't married to. Or, in some cases, wasn't yet married to. That's not a new thing, but it has only recently won public acceptance. I never felt I had to have public acceptance. I don't think anyone should do anything just because someone else approves or disapproves. I think people should think for themselves. I also feel that people should rethink traditional ways of life if new ways seem to work better.

I'm not pursuing eternal youth, but I don't think age should be a barrier blocking my way to happiness. At fifty-one, I seem to desire sex as much as I did at twenty. Fortunately for my marriage, the lady I happen to desire happens to be my wife.

I have married a woman thirteen years younger than I am. I see nothing wrong with that. It is sort of traditional for a man to desire a younger woman, but I didn't desire this lady because she's younger than I am, but because she's the lady she is.

She does help me feel young, however. A lot of what I have done is new to her. Doing these things again, with her, makes me feel young again. I do things with youthful enthusiasm. I try not to make her feel old. She says I do not. She says she can't keep up with me.

It may not be traditional, but it is now accepted when an older woman is interested in, goes with, lives with, or marries a younger man. Why not? Why should age matter? It is the way you feel about a lover or a mate that matters. It is how you feel that matters. If you feel young, you are young.

Conversely, if you are interested in an older person, remember that it's the way you feel that matters, not the years.

I also have had three children, one with my first wife and two with my second. I don't know if I will have any with my third. If my wife wants one, we will. So far she says she doesn't. You may think I'm too old, but I feel young enough. Jockey Bill Shoemaker just had his first child at fifty-three.

My children are grown up or growing up. Aside from the kids on my shows, I have had teen-agers in my home in recent years, and they have helped me stay young. I try to talk to them and listen to them, and they keep me current.

If you want to stay young, you have to know what the young are thinking. If you want to keep up with the world, you have to keep current. If you don't want to be old before your time, you have to do something about it.

In the chapters to come, I'll talk about

the things you can do. I'll lean on expert advice whenever it is logical to do so.

I'm not going to give you a lot of diets or long lists of dos and don'ts. I'm not going to design a detailed program for you to follow. You won't have to keep a daily diary.

Informally, I'm going to suggest some things that might be helpful to you. If you take from this what attracts and interests you, I suspect it will help you look better and younger, feel better and younger, and stay younger and be happier.

2

Thinking Young

Nostalgia is "in" these days. A lot of shows are devoted to the 1930s, '40s, '50s, and even the '60s. Broadway and Hollywood musical hits of recent years have centered on the life and music of these past periods. Television programs like "Happy Days" and "Laverne and Shirley" center on life in another era. Some radio stations play nothing but "oldies" of other eras. Concerts devoted to performers of the '40s and '50s are popular.

In the 1970s I was talked into taking a *Good Ol' Rock 'n' Roll* review into the Las Vegas Hilton. I was surprised at how well we did with it, and I've toured successfully with similar shows from time to time since. People love to remember the stars of their youth and the songs they grew up with and romanced to.

There's nothing wrong with this. I grew up in the 1940s and I'm still fond of the music of the big-band era, of Benny Goodman, Harry James, Tommy Dorsey, and Glenn Miller; of Frank Sinatra, Dick Haymes, Bob Eberle, Helen O'Connell, Helen Forrest, and Peggy Lee. Obviously, I'm also partial to the music of the 1950s, when "American Bandstand" started. I have a big record collection and often listen to the music of this era. But I listen to today's music more.

Yesterday is gone. It's startling to stop and think that the music I listen to on a local radio station devoted to the big-band era is forty years old. But we all relate to the music of our youth.

I suppose the teen-age years are the most traumatic of our lives. We begin to grow apart from our parents and start to do things on our own. We have vivid experiences. Dating, for one. First sex, for another. First job, for another. We form our philosophies of life. Our personalities take shape. We will change with the years and with different experiences, but I believe the basis for the person we will be is shaped most drastically when we are teen-agers.

I never use the term "puppy love" or

put down "first love" because I believe it has an impact on us that lasts all our lives. We usually remember well the first girl or boy we went with, the first one we went to bed with. If it was a good experience, it is a happy memory. If it was a bad one, it is an unhappy memory. Either way, it tends to have a lasting impact beyond many others that come later.

I married my high school sweetheart. I think we married because we had been going together for a long time — or at least it seemed a long time at the time — and it was expected of us. We just sort of assumed we would marry after a while. We did not have the depth of feeling for each other or understanding of each other we needed to make the marriage work. It did not last forever, but it lasted almost ten years and brought us a wonderful child. The marriage was not the best experience I've had, but it was far from the worst.

All our feelings are magnified when we are young because we are going through experiences for the first time and haven't had other experiences to compare them with. When we break up with the first love of our life, we think the world will end. We think we will never love again. Time teaches most of us otherwise. We find we can love many people in many ways. Most of us have several romances. Many of us marry more than once. Too many, maybe. The lucky ones find a depth of feeling and understanding in romance that makes for a lasting marriage.

As we grow older, the music changes. The big-band era of my youth lasted a few years after World War II and gave way to the rock 'n' roll rage of the 1950s. I grew up listening to "The Make-Believe Ballroom" on radio and wanting to be a disc jockey, playing big-band records. I was still young when I started on "American Bandstand" on television, playing rock 'n' roll records.

I don't suppose any music of the young ever was put down by the old as hard as rock 'n' roll was. It was a drastic departure from the swing music of the big bands. Few thought rock 'n' roll would last. It did. The people who grew up with rock 'n' roll remember it as affectionately as those of us who grew up with the swing era. We tend to associate the most memorable moments of our life with the songs and records that were popular in our youth.

Frank Sinatra has endured for forty years because he has a talent that has endured and because many of us associate certain records of his with important times in our lives. He has been a part of our lives longer than any other public personality, perhaps, although a George Burns, a James Stewart, or a Bette Davis has similar memories for us. When a Bing Crosby or Jack Benny dies, it is as though a member of our family has died.

The music changed in the 1960s. It changed again in the '70s. But the changes grew out of rock 'n' roll. Just as rock 'n' roll grew out of swing. You don't think so? Just listen. Put on some of the rhythm and blues records made by the black artists of the swing era and see how close they come to the Elvis Presley or Jerry Lee Lewis records that followed.

You can follow this line through to the Beatles. Elton John and the Bee Gees grew out of the Beatles. We grow. We change and grow. But we do not have to grow older.

I think we have to change if we are going to stay young. "American Bandstand" began before the rock 'n' roll era. I knew nothing about the new music when I started with the show. I learned. I listened to the kids and their music, and I learned. Or the show would have failed.

Most people have tunnel vision. They have built-in blinders. They don't see the world around them because they don't look around them. They see only their own world and themselves. This applies to kids as well as to older people.

If you talk to a high school kid, he'll tell you how he sees things. He sure as hell won't tell you how his parents and teachers see things. If you talk to a businessman, he'll tell you all his troubles. He sure won't tell you about his customers' troubles. Most people don't listen well. One of the secrets to staying young is not talking to the young but listening to the young.

If you're a listener, it will work to your advantage. If you try to tell a kid what you think or where he's wrong, he'll turn off. He'll say you're wrong. And he'll be right. He'll wonder how you could have lived so long and gotten so dumb. But if you listen to him, you can learn something about him and get smart. Here's where the collapse in communication between parents and their children can be reconstructed. There doesn't have to be a generation gap. If you show an interest in your child, in really listening to his or her point of view, your child may listen to you. When you show an interest in and really listen to anyone, that person may find you interesting and listen to you.

In a sense, we're all salesmen. We're trying to sell ourselves and our points of view. We want the world to see us as we see ourselves. The smart salesman listens to the customer. He finds out what makes him tick. He finds out how to talk to him. You can't talk to everyone alike and expect to get the same response from everyone. But if you're interested in people, and dig into them, you'll dig up stuff you can use.

I don't think you can fake it. Especially with kids. Kids can spot a phony in

five seconds. You have to be really interested. You have to be willing to consider
what they think, and you have to be willing to change the way you think if you
see they are making good points. You
have to be willing to change. It'll keep
you young in the process.

As the music has changed, I have
changed. Kids change. Every generation
has new and different attitudes. Listening to them and their music, I have kept
up. Keeping up, I have kept "American
Bandstand" on the air. I know it won't be
on forever. In time, television viewers tire
of the best shows. The most popular
shows have come and gone. An "I Love
Lucy" lingers on in reruns, but not in
prime time and not with anywhere near
the audience it once had. I'm proud that
"American Bandstand" has lasted as long
as it has. Few shows ever lasted as long.

I love today's music. I may not be into
the latest things yet. I don't know if
they'll last. But I'll listen. Maybe I'll never
really love them. But I'll give them every
chance. We can't all love everything. But
we can give everything a chance.

I just don't understand people who
say they haven't liked any new music
since the 1940s, who listen only to big-
band records, who go only to swing-era
shows. I don't think they ever really listened to the music of recent decades or
went to shows featuring the stars of
these eras. It's like saying *Gone With the*

Wind was such a great movie you didn't want to see *Star Wars* or won't see *The Empire Strikes Back*.

I constantly run into people who tell me that their high school or college days were the best times of their lives, whose conversation consists of remembering the bash at the frat house when drunken Charlie rolled down the stairs. I say, "Wow, I forgot that a hundred years ago." Sure those were good times. But I've had a lot of good times since. I'm having good times today. I can remember yesterday, but I don't want to spend all my time doing it. I'd rather enjoy today and look forward to tomorrow.

I think it's sad that our deepest friendships are made in high school or college. I suppose it's only natural to feel close to the people with whom we shared those traumatic growing-up years, those first experiences, but people change, and frequently the only thing we have in common with the friends of our youth are memories. I'd like to think we could make even deeper and more enduring friendships with the people we meet and like in our lives today. I think I have.

Explaining "American Bandstand," I say, "We play the music, the kids dance, and America watches." It is almost that simple. We bring on the popular performers of the day. They lip-synch their hits to their records. We never have kidded anyone about that. There is no way we could reproduce the sounds of the records live on our show week after week and be able to afford to do the show, and it is these sounds the kids want to hear. We also talk to the stars. The kids in the viewing audience can relate to the stars this way. And we talk to the kids on our show. They express what those in the viewing audience are thinking.

There have always been more adults in the viewing audience. Watching shows that deal with the youth of today is one way that adults can learn what the kids are thinking, how they look at life, and how their way may differ from the way we look at life today. I think I was lucky to fall into a life that required me to relate to the young. It has helped keep me current, keep me young.

Those of us who put together the show learned early on to limit the kids on the show to those between the ages of fourteen and twenty. We found that kids under fourteen were too self-conscious on camera, too giddy and difficult to control, and those over twenty felt too sophisticated to really relax and enjoy themselves, and it showed on camera. There are exceptions, of course, but we had to draw the line somewhere, and we found the ages of fourteen to twenty provided the most typical "teen-agers." And those fifteen, sixteen, and seventeen were best of all.

In any event, I have dealt primarily with kids fourteen to twenty on the show. I was not yet thirty when I first went on with the show, but even that was many years older than the oldest kids on the show. I wasn't old enough to be a father figure to them. Most people likened me to an older brother. I don't know. I know I didn't try to be anything like that. I tried to be a friend. I think you can be a friend to someone a lot younger than you are. As well as to someone a lot older. I know I tried, and I think it worked. I was sincerely interested in finding out what the young people thought so that I could find out what would make my show work. I think my sincerity showed through. They accepted me.

Twenty-some years later, I *am* old enough to be their father. I have been a father to three teen-agers of my own. And I have used in my life the lessons I learned on the show. I still try to keep current with the kids in order to keep the show current, but I do it for more than that. I am not entirely a calculating person. I am an interested person. I am interested in people and in life. I think I still relate to the teen-agers on the show and still am accepted by them because the sincerity of my interest shows through. I think they still accept me as their friend because I still want to be friends with them. I don't really want to be a big brother. I am too old for that now, anyway. I don't want to be their father. I have enough on my hands being a father to my own kids. I do want to be friends with the kids on my show.

A father can't really be a friend to his kids, though I think there is a feeling of friendship between my kids and me. I always wanted to go places and do things with my kids, although I fell into the same trap as most fathers in that I was too often too busy. I think my kids knew I wanted to be with them and do things with them, and I swung it as often as I could. But, as a father, I often had to guide them and discipline them and try to teach them a good set of values. Along with their mother, of course. I had to rely largely on my own upbringing and my own experiences. But I honestly tried to listen to them and understand what they were thinking. I tried to relate to the lives they were leading, which were different from the life I led as I grew up.

I don't pretend my kids are perfect. I think they're pretty good. I did my best with them. Most of us do our best and hope for the best. I do think sometimes we could do better. We could talk less and listen more. I don't think the rules we were asked to live by when we were young have to apply to the young of today. Oh, some of the rules, yes. Rules relating to basic honesty, for example. Rules for showing respect to others. But,

I think the young feel freer to express themselves and be themselves today, and we should encourage this. We can learn to stay young by applying that thinking to ourselves.

I don't think we can understand them unless we encourage them to be themselves. I always have encouraged my kids and the kids on my show to be themselves. I always asked them what they thought about this or that and asked them what they thought of my generation, and I listened so that I could try to understand them and their thinking. I never tried to impose my views on them, but if they asked me, I told them what I thought. There was an exchange there, and I think this is what is missing when we talk of a generation gap.

As the years have gone by I have tried to talk to the kids about the music they enjoy, the dances they enjoy, the things they like and don't like in life, what they think of life and what they hope to do with their lives. I think in many ways their ideals are better than ours. Over the years, their work in the Peace Corps, their opposition to war, their freeing themselves of many of the hangups we had about sex reflect this and have proved a positive influence in the world. I haven't always agreed with them, but I have grown with them and have changed my views on many things. In so doing, I am younger for it.

I have tried to learn the language of the young so that I can understand what the young are saying. I like to know the language of the day, and it keeps changing. I don't use whatever the current vernacular is. For one thing, it changes too fast and I would be dated fast. For another, I'd never be comfortable using it. It would make me look foolish. Any older person who tries this is making a mistake. I don't put on a pose that I'm "hip." Kids can see right through those masks. But I believe I am current in that I hear young people and know what they're saying. Being young is not acting young. It's *thinking* young. And trying to understand what the young are thinking.

It goes past teen-agers, of course. You have to listen to college kids. They're really not kids by the time they get to college, of course. They're young adults, but their thinking is fresh and free. They're on the brink of the lives they will live as adults, and they're really concerned about what those lives will be. The college crowd often is the most influential in any community, in any country. They're rebellious. They're ready to reshape the world. They don't think we did such a good job with the world, and they're right. They might not do any better, but at least they haven't given up, the way many of us have. They are ready to do their best, which many of us no longer are.

I don't think many of us who are forty
or fifty years old now think that our participation in the conflict in Vietnam was
entirely justified, but most of us just did
not think about it a lot, or do anything
about it at the time we were there. And I
think we would still be there if the young
hadn't acted for us. I haven't approved of
all the protests and demonstrations by
the young in recent years, but I think
they were right about many wrongs. And
I'm glad they fought for those things they
believed in. Most of us old folks have
benefited from many changes the young
have effected.

If we listen to the young, we can learn
a lot. And we shouldn't just listen. We
should allow them to lead us where they
have taken the lead on issues on which
we agree. When we are moved to do so,
we should act. We should participate
with them. Action keeps us young. Participation keeps us young. We let ourselves be old and out of touch with the
times when we sit back and let the
young do all the living and benefit by all
the changes. Our lives aren't perfect; they
can be improved. This applies whether
we are "successful" or not.

What is success, anyway? Is it gaining
fame or making a lot of money? I don't
think so. I've had a certain amount of
fame and made a fair amount of money,
and I don't think I'd be happy if that was
all I had. If I couldn't pay my bills, I'd be

unhappy, sure. If I considered myself one who hadn't done anything, I'd also be unhappy. But I think it is living life to the fullest that makes me happy, and I feel I'm happy. I enjoy life. I look forward to every day. I think you can be happy only if you live for today. I know I do not live like I did yesterday.

I do not speak the kids' language of today, but I understand it and relate to it and can carry on a conversation with someone who uses it. I do not dress like a teen-ager. I think the man or woman who does this tends to make a fool of himself or herself. But I read magazines and know what the styles are and dress as young as I dare.

I read everything from the trashiest teen magazines to the best business magazines. I try to keep up with current trends and thoughts. I know what is expected and accepted today and what is not. If I don't like something, I don't do it. But if I find merit in something new, I'm not afraid to try it. I can change with the times, and I think that is important to anyone who wants to stay young. I learn new things every day. I find I accept a lot of these things. And I can deal with the rest.

When I was young, it was really rare for a guy and gal to live together before marriage. It was frowned on. I'd have found it difficult to do. In recent years, it's become more accepted. I've looked at

it and thought about it and come to accept it. I think it may be a good idea for
people who are unsure about themselves
in one way or another. I suppose it depends on the degree of commitment
you're willing to make to another person.
I am sure you're risking a lot of unhap-
piness if you make a marriage you're not
sure of.

I do believe in marriage. The last lady
I lived with I did marry. We decided we
were ready. We decided we not only
loved each other but we could live with
each other. These are two different
things. Living with someone, you may
find you don't want to live with her the
rest of your life. I think it's wise to find
out if you can live with someone before
you marry that person. You may not
agree. You do owe it to yourself to think
about it.

One thing that has helped my wife
and me so far is the new openness between the sexes. I don't know why, but
only in recent years has there been a lot
of emphasis put on men and women
talking freely and frankly to each other. It
seems to me a lot of marriages broke
down because husband and wife
couldn't or wouldn't communicate their
true feelings to each other. They had
roles to play, and they played them. If
they were dissatisfied, they kept it to
themselves until the emotional buildup
within them led to explosions.

The traditional roles have broken down. Women still have to carry the babies, but men now participate at the birth of their children. They share in the experience as much as possible. They should, because they share in the children. Husbands diaper and change their children. They can't breast-feed, but they can bottle-feed and often take over the middle-of-the-night feedings. I wish I'd seen my babies born. I did do the other stuff. Why not?

We're equal. But only in recent years have we really realized this. Women are still striving for full equality. It's hard to believe that it was only about 60 years ago that women got the vote. Well, it's less than 150 years since we abolished slavery. Some people would still like to have slaves. Some would like to keep the ladies in the kitchen. Or the bedroom. I want them there. But, also, elsewhere. I want my woman to be wherever she wants to be.

As it happens, my wife, Kari, works side by side with me. She knows my business and contributes to it. I respect her instincts and listen to her suggestions. I had children with my previous marriages, but right now Kari and I do not have anyone else living full-time in our home. We are free to work together and travel together. Having had two failures in marriage, I am not foolish enough to think that the success of my present marriage is assured, but it has been successful so far, and we are working at keeping it so. We have open minds and listen to each other's thoughts and respect each other's feelings. We are trying to be youthful and keep our marriage youthful. I think that at the least we are giving it a good chance.

I have learned a lot about women in recent years and am learning more all the time simply because I feel free to talk to women and ask them about their feelings as I never did before. I am told by women the same is true for them with men. It is unbelievable that in this day and age a man and woman can't be friends without some sort of sexual involvement or implication. There are some old fogeys who feel the sexual difference between the sexes is all that matters.

One of the new developments in recent years has been the Marriage Encounter experience. I cannot speak with any expertise about this because I've never been involved with it. My wife and I never have felt the need. But, if we did, I think we'd try it. A lot of married couples have told me they've gotten a lot out of it. I think wherever you feel a need for something, you should try to find something to fill it. When you're young, you try all sorts of new things. Trying new things helps you to stay young.

If you feel you'd like the social life,

join a social club or a dance club. If you can't dance, take lessons and learn to dance. If you're single, join a singles club. If you like to play tennis or golf but never get around to it, join a tennis club or a golf club. Or a swim club. Or any kind of club that appeals to you. Don't be afraid to try these things. If you don't like one, try another. The big thing is to try. Don't be afraid you'll feel out of place. Chances are you'll find your place. I'll give you some expert tips on the way to dress in the "Dressing Right" chapter. The important thing is to give different things a chance.

If something attracts you about *est*, Transcendental Meditation, the Human Potential Movement, or any other program, try it. If you like it, get into it. I'm interested in hypnotism and self-hypnosis. I took a mind-control course once and found myself fascinated by it. I found we do not control our minds as well as we can. Once we set our minds on something, we lock them in place. We always see things in the same way. We can control our minds, however. We can look at things from different perspectives. Things may have changed. Or we may perceive them to have changed because we are looking at them in a changed way. We can open our minds.

Hypnotism may be the way. If a football team can "psych" itself up, why can't you? Our minds remain mysteries to us.

Through hypnotism we may open up our minds and solve some mysteries. One of my sons suffered for years from nightmares that left him shaken when he woke up. In desperation, having exhausted all normal medical cures, he agreed to see a hypnotist, Arthur Ellen. He worked what seems to me to have been a miraculous cure on the boy, in one visit. That was many years ago. My son has never had another bad nightmare experience.

Ellen says, "I do not make miracles. I cannot cure you of your problems. What I can do with hypnotism is free you to help yourself. And if a cure can be found, you can find it. I do not put people 'under.' No qualified therapeutic hypnotist does. You are awake and conscious of what is happening to you. But in the hypnotized state your mind becomes clear. Bad memories, fears, or other things you may have repressed are freed to rise to the surface. You can see them, consider them, deal with them. I cannot make you better than you are. A person who cannot sing in tune cannot become a great singer. But I can free you to become the best person you can be. I can clear your mind so you can concentrate on doing any task the best you can."

I think that's what we all want — to be the best we can be, to do the best we can do. Hypnotism may or may not be the way. It is one way we can try. It appeals to me. It may not appeal to you. If not, try another way. Look for something that appeals to you. Don't try something because it's popular, but because it appeals to you. Get interested in what's going on around you. Look into anything that interests you, even if it's unpopular. Don't laugh off things because others laugh at them. That's the old way. The young way is to look into things before deciding about them. Based on my experience, I'm not likely to laugh at hypnotism as something that can help people.

I don't go to a psychiatrist, but I don't look down on people who do. If I felt troubled, if I felt my mind was mixed up, I wouldn't hesitate to go to one. Not because it's the Hollywood thing to do, but because it's the smart thing to do. Find professional help whenever you feel you need it. It doesn't matter what others think. It's what you think that matters. It's old hat to dismiss psychiatrists as "shrinks."

Many people feel yoga works wonders for them. Many meditate daily. They feel this freshens them both physically and mentally. There may be nothing new about this, but it is new to those who try it for the first time. Trying new things, we stay young. It is the youthful thing to do. It opens up our lives and expands our horizons.

You should talk with and listen not

only to the young but to anyone who is into anything new or anyone you meet who has had experiences you have not. I try to learn from the actors and actresses, directors and producers, advertising men and businessmen I deal with every day, not only those in my profession but everyone I encounter from other professions. You owe it to yourself to find out about anything that may fit into your life or the life style you'd like to lead.

Sometimes we work side by side with someone we do not really know. Often we dismiss suggestions made by a newcomer. The smart thing to do is to find out about the people we work with, find out what they are thinking, consider their ideas. We tend to find something that works for us, and we stick to it. But we might find something that works better. A young comedian finds a routine, a series of sketches — "shtick," as we call it — that works and sticks to it. For the most part, he will find it will not work forever. If he does not vary his "shtick," the audience will tire of it. Often, he doesn't understand why. It always worked, why not now? He is thinking old. If he were thinking young, he would be looking for routines that were fresh. If he came up with creative routines in the beginning, he could do so now. But he does not. He is old now.

"American Bandstand" is one thing. It appeals to a wide audience range, including teen-agers. There always are new teen-agers coming along. The show is new to them. We change the show as teen-agers change. We change the music as the music changes. The "$20,000 Pyramid" was another thing. I talked to the people who played the game and watched the show to find out what interested them in the show. The money contestants could win was important, of course. Everyone wants to win money. But I do not believe greed drove our contestants and fans. They knew few would win anything big. Those in the audience couldn't win. I think the secret to the success of these shows is that it is fun to see ordinary people trying to win extraordinary prizes. Naturally, they are overjoyed if they win, disappointed if they lose; but we all root for them, though it won't put a penny in our pockets. It is fun for us, as it is for them. So these shows stress the fun part as well as the prizes.

With my production company, I always try new things. I have learned to try new things. I have made mistakes on new things. Hey, you are hearing from a first-class jackass! I hate to tell you how many giant hit records I have missed or turned down. Using my infallible instinct, I was the one who advised Bobby Darin not to release "Mack the Knife." Probably his biggest hit! I took one look at the hula hoop and told them to go fly a kite. Well, it *didn't* last. About a billion bucks worth of business down the road, you don't see them much anymore! You live, and if you're smart, you learn. Now, if someone brings me something new, I take a long look at it. I keep an open mind. No one can predict what will work in this world. No one knows what games will catch on, what gimmicks will hit. No one knows which songs will make it, what the trends will be. But if you're youthful in your approach to things, you may guess right sometimes.

If they say a certain show won't work, I want to try to make it work. If they say such and such never has been done before, I want to try to do it. I'm fortunate that I'm in a business that is wide open and loves long shots. They said rock 'n' roll was dead, so I created a rock 'n' roll revival show that's broken house attendance records for years. In this case something old became something new. We produced "Elvis" in 1979. A lot of people were skeptical about it, but ABC-TV devoted an entire night of prime time to it — three hours. The other networks threw the Academy Award winning movies *Gone With the Wind* and *One Flew Over the Cuckoo's Nest* against us. Most thought we would be wiped out. Instead, we wiped them out. We do not always win. No one does. But we can try. And keep trying.

Don't be afraid to look for new concepts in your business or your life. Pretend you are back at the beginning. Try to recapture your youthful enthusiasm. Seek new things that will breathe new life into your activities. Try to reshape them with the same enthusiasm you had when you shaped them back at the beginning. Make a new beginning. Make a fresh start. Talk to people who are doing something different. See if perhaps you wouldn't be wise to do different.

If you have a secretary, sit down with her sometime and ask her about her job and her life, what she likes and doesn't like, what she does and what she would like to do. Try to look at her job as she does. You may gain the information that will enable you to enable her to do a better job for you, one that will make her happier and make you happier. If you are interested in her work, she will be interested in yours. Make contact with the people you work with. Make them a part of the team. Don't accept traditional roles and relationships anywhere in your life.

If someone tries to sell you insurance, listen to his proposal, but also ask him about his job. It may be that you'll want to try selling insurance someday. At the least, you'll get an understanding of what an insurance salesman does so that you can deal with his and other insurance people's proposals more intelligently. Ask about and find out about the jobs people do around you so that you can understand their work better and have a better understanding of what to expect from them. Be as curious as a kid.

Try new things. So you like a restaurant and eat there once a week. You'll never know if you like another one just as well or better if you don't try others. So you like a thick steak and a baked potato. Try the fish and rice sometimes. Try something you haven't tried. Pick a different thing off the menu each time for a while. Perhaps there is something there you haven't had since you were young. You didn't like it then. You might now. The young try everything. Try frog's legs. Or snails. Or raw fish. You might be surprised. You stay young if you keep trying things.

"Hey, I found something new," you'll say to people.

So you go to Hawaii every year for your vacation. It's beautiful and you love it. But try Alaska sometime. It's beautiful in a different way. You may like it even better. At the worst, it will be different, interesting, a new experience. So you like gambling and go to Las Vegas from time to time. Try Tahoe sometime. It has the same slots, tables, and shows. Plus majestic mountains and a lovely lake. Or Reno, an Old West town. Or, now, Atlantic City, an old resort town with a new look. Any good travel agent can give you good guidance.

I always look for new places to see. When Kari and I take vacations, we pick new places. If we've been somewhere, we want to go somewhere else. The days and nights seem longer in new places. Everything you see and do is different. Each day and each night is a new adventure. So you can't afford Alaska or Hawaii, Atlantic City or Las Vegas. Try Chicago or New Orleans or San Francisco. Or the next town over.

Try an ocean cruise, short or long, here or there. Or a train ride. How long has it been since you were on a train? Or even a bus ride? Many of the trains and buses these days have scenic tours with glass-enclosed cabins through which to see the country and long stops at fascinating places in this country or other countries. Open up your life and get a fresh look at life as others live it.

See your own town as you've never seen it before. Have you any idea how many New Yorkers have never been to the Statue of Liberty, how many Angelenos have never been to the Hollywood Bowl? More have not than have been, I'm told. The world is at your fingertips. Reach out for it with the same curiosity the baby shows as he begins to crawl and is anxious to reach, touch, even taste everything in his world.

We tend to drift into ruts. We curl up comfortably. And age away. We stop going out to eat. We have meatloaf every

Monday. We have the same eight to ten things month after month. We have a television set, so we watch it every night. We don't talk to one another. We don't have friends over to talk or play cards. Or we play cards every Tuesday. We never read a book anymore. We don't have time. But we turn on TV. We stop going to the movies. Or plays. Or concerts. Or dances. Or ballgames. We like them, but we've been. We're tired, and it's too much trouble.

If we think of ourselves as tired, we will be. If we think of something as too much trouble, it will be. But if we get up and go, we'll find there's a lot of energy left in us and a lot of life to be lived that we haven't been living. That's what staying young is — living life to its fullest.

Do things on impulse. Scoop the family up for a picnic. Find a baby-sitter and take the wife to a motel. (Or the husband. Women can act on impulse, too.) Make a date with your wife or husband. If you don't have one, find a date. Do something different.

You'll come home and say, "Wasn't that a great movie!" or, "Wasn't that a lousy movie, but wasn't it fun to be holding hands and eating popcorn in the theater again!" "Wasn't that a great game?" Or, "I haven't danced like that in years!" You may be worn out, but I guarantee you, you'll feel refreshed. You'll feel young again. You will be young again.

You will be thinking young. You're up and about. You're on the move. You look forward to each day because you are looking at the world in a new way.

3

Resisting
Stress

I'm a workaholic. It's not good, but there it is. It isn't too bad if you've learned how to handle it. I think I have. I think my work keeps me young. I don't ever want to retire. I don't think you should. But if you want to retire, or you have retired, find something to do. Find a hobby. Collect stamps, start painting. Take up photography or bird watching, anything that attracts you. Find out how you can help people. Volunteer at a hospital. Become a Big Brother. Enlist in the Scouts. Find something.

It's when you have nothing to do that you age away, that you start to live in the past. You have to have something to look forward to every day. No matter how old you are, you have to live every day like the young do.

I come from an average middle-class background in Mount Vernon, New York, a Westchester County suburb of New York City. My father was a salesman. My mother was a housewife. I had an older brother, Bradley, who graduated from high school in 1943, enlisted in the Air Force, and was killed in combat during the Battle of the Bulge late in 1944. I was fifteen years old and devastated. I still miss him.

My family lived in an apartment. The walls of my room were covered with movie stars' pictures I'd sent away for. I always liked movies and show business. I liked to listen to the radio and to music. This was before television, of course. I listened to Martin Block's "Make-Believe Ballroom" every afternoon and Art Ford's "Milkman's Matinee" until late at night. I also liked Arthur Godfrey, Steve Allen, the talkers. After my parents took me to see a live broadcast of the Garry Moore and Jimmy Durante radio show, I wanted to do something like that for a living.

I took my parents' suggestion to join the high school dramatic club. Here, I gained a lot of confidence in performing in public. I looked into what colleges had radio schools and wound up at Syracuse University. We had just moved upstate to

Utica. My uncle owned a newspaper in the area, had just opened a radio station, and offered my dad a job as sales manager. He took it and we went.

I asked for and got a summer job at WRUN in Utica. At first I did the dirty jobs, odd jobs. Then I got to pinch-hit for a vacationing announcer on the station's FM outlet. I started with the weather. Then I went on to do the news and station breaks on the AM outlet. When I got to Syracuse, I volunteered for the campus station, WAER-FM. In time, I was doing not only newscasts but a disc jockey show and even a talk show.

By the time I was a senior at Syracuse, I was applying for jobs at local stations. I landed one working weekends at WOLF. Soon I was full-time, forty hours a week at a dollar an hour. I did newscasts and played records.

After graduation, I returned to WRUN. But I soon decided I wasn't wise working for my father and my uncle. I had to get out on my own. I got a job with WKTV, the only TV station in Utica at the time. I even changed my name to Dick Clay to separate my identification from my father, who was the best-known Dick Clark in Utica.

I replaced Bob Earle, who was going on to bigger and better things. He later became emcee of the network "GE College Bowl." I was amazed at the way he did the news without looking at notes or "idiot cards." He taught me to tape my newscast, wear a concealed earphone, and hear it as I said it. I had a foot-pedal device to stop and go. Doing the news, I developed a friendly, conversational style. I was successful. At twenty, I was ready to take on the world.

I auditioned at WFIL radio-TV in Philadelphia. I was tested with tongue-twister copy, but my tape-recorder trick turned the trick. I passed the test and started with the radio station. I began with station breaks. In time I got to do commercials and newscasts. I even acted a few parts in radio dramas the station did. When the station stopped taking most of its programs from ABC and decided to do most of its shows locally, I got to do a DJ show, "Dick Clark's Caravan of Music," four hours every weekday afternoon.

In Philadelphia I went back to being Dick Clark. The music they had me playing wasn't Dick Clark's kind of music, but I didn't have much to say about it. I got extra money for the commercials I did on the show, and I got by.

I auditioned for and got the chance to do commercials for other companies. I did so well for Schaefer Beer in Philadelphia that they had me commute to New York to do their beer plugs on a weekly wrestling show they had there. One night Rudy Schaefer saw me and told them to take me off. He said the kid was too young to drink their product. Another guy got the job and made a lot of money at it. My youthful look hasn't always been an asset. They wouldn't let me do the news in Philadelphia because they said I looked too young to know what was going on in the world. If some people say I look thirty at fifty, can you imagine what I looked like at twenty-five?

I did drink beer, though. I had drunk quite a bit one night when I had to do a finance company commercial. I was supposed to say, "You folks up there in Frankford." Instead I said, "You fucks up there in Frankford." The fellows in the studio fell on the floor all around me. I thought my career would fall apart around me — but it didn't. We all make mistakes. The fact is, no one called. I guess no one was listening, at least not closely!

The TV station replaced its afternoon movie with a show called "Bob Horn's Bandstand." The station had a library of short musical films, and Bob played these and interviewed musical guests. The show adopted a format of playing records and bringing in kids to dance to them. It was not Bob's idea to bring in a co-host, Lee Stewart, to provide comedy relief, but the station did. The co-hosts could have been better, but the show became a hit. They even changed the name of my radio show to "Dick Clark's Bandstand" and brought in Bob Horn at the start and finish to promote his TV show on my radio show.

Horn had good ideas, but neither he nor Stewart was a vivid visual personality. Eventually, Stewart was sent to another show. Then Horn was fired. The show was turned over to me. I had done it as a summer replacement and took it over full-time in July of 1956. I did not make up the show, but I think I made it the show it became. I got closer to the kids and I got closer to what they liked. They rated the records and the stars. We got greater stars on the show. I got to where I was a good judge of what and who were going to be big, and we introduced a lot of winners on the show.

We had on Jerry Lee Lewis, James Brown, Bill Haley, Paul Anka, Bobby Darin, Fats Domino, Frankie Avalon, Chuck Berry, Connie Francis, the Everly Brothers, everyone who was big with the kids in those days except Elvis Presley, who didn't do such shows, and Ricky Nelson, who did only his own show. We had some of the same kids coming right to the studio from school to dance every day so the audience could identify with them. Some of those kids became stars of sorts themselves. A lot of adults disliked the music and feared for their children. But if a lot of parents disliked the show, their children liked it, so it lasted.

I went to the network in New York

and pleaded for a trial run nationally. We got four weeks in August of 1957 and have been on nationally ever since. In March of 1964 we moved the show to Los Angeles. While it is now on only Saturday afternoons, for many years it was on every weekday afternoon and for a while even on Saturday nights in prime time. I was on the cover of *TV Guide* and all the major television and teen-age magazines frequently. I was the subject of a "This Is Your Life" TV show with Ralph Edwards, and my wife and I were interviewed by Edward R. Murrow on "Person to Person."

I've crisscrossed the country with *The Dick Clark Caravan of Stars* and still host *The Good Ol' Rock 'n' Roll* revue in Las Vegas, Reno, Tahoe, and Atlantic City, and at state fairs and in major theme parks. I've acted in three movies — *Because They Are Young, The Young Doctors*, and *Killers Three* — I don't know why they didn't call it *The Young Killers* — as well as in many television dramas. For more than seven years, I hosted the "The $20,000 Pyramid" on TV.

Our production company is involved in television and motion pictures and personal appearance productions. We have the rights to several major books. We currently are producing half a dozen motion pictures for theatrical release worldwide, two films for television, a

syndicated radio show in the United
States, Canada, Australia, and New Zea-
land.

We operate a concert division pro-
moting all kinds of talent. On television,
annually, we do the "American Music
Awards," the "Academy of Country
Music Awards," and "New Year's Rockin'
Eve."

At one time I wrote a syndicated
newspaper column. All the time I am
getting into things I have no business
getting into. I've just gotten into the fight
to stop people putting oil wells into and
polluting Santa Monica Bay. I have interests outside my work, and I can't seem to
avoid deep involvements.

I may not be the busiest guy in the
world, but I'm busy. Some guys go
harder, but I go coast to coast every week
or two, and I am always on the go. I
seem to be juggling ninety-seven balls in
the air all the time. I always wind up saying why not this, that, and this, too; why
not three more and make it an even
hundred? And then, why not a hundred
and three? I'm sure a lot of you feel the
same way. Well, hell, we're lucky to have
plenty to do. It would be one heck of a
lot worse if we had too little to do. If you
don't have enough to do or have nothing
to do, you're unlucky, and you'd better
start looking for things to do to keep you
going, to keep you young. I don't think

people die from overwork. I think they die from boredom.

That's a simplification, of course. I think you can work too hard and wear yourself out and suffer from high blood pressure and hypertension and heart trouble, but there are ways of dealing with these things. I don't think there is any way to make boredom any better except getting busy. I think that having work we want to do keeps us in the present and keeps us young, and that not having enough to do puts us in the past and makes us feel old.

I work because I want to. I was lucky enough to find something I wanted to do that I could do, and I wake up every morning looking forward to going to work. I think the worst thing in the world is drifting into some job you dislike so much you hate to get up in the morning and spending all day watching the clock in hope the day will soon be done. It has to be horrible to wake up with nothing to do and nowhere to go.

I don't work for the money or the fame. I'd be lying if I said I didn't like the spotlight and didn't like the rewards, but I've had all I really need of both and by this time am hungry for neither. Twenty years ago, I had made all the money anyone could ever need. I'm not the richest guy in the business by any means, but there's big money in the entertainment business, and anyone who is successful in it can make it. I've invested my money carefully and still have a lot of it.

After a while, prominence pales. After a while, you'd prefer to go out in the world without attracting attention and being asked for autographs and being unable to enjoy what you're doing. I guess when you get right down to it, I'm driven by the desire simply to be successful, no matter the other pluses and minuses. I've been successful, but I want to stay successful. I don't ever want to be "washed up."

I've done some good things, but some of the things I've done haven't been the greatest. I'd like to do things better, to do new and better things. I think most people in most businesses feel the same way in the beginning, but you can lose your ambition, and reversals and disappointments can sap your spirit. If that's happened to you, buck up and begin anew.

One of the great things about being young is that you haven't yet had many reversals or deep disappointments; anything you want is still possible. Well, try to recapture that youthful enthusiasm. Give it another go. Take another shot at the brass ring. It will be like being born again, young again!

Depending on what we have had going for us at our offices, we have had

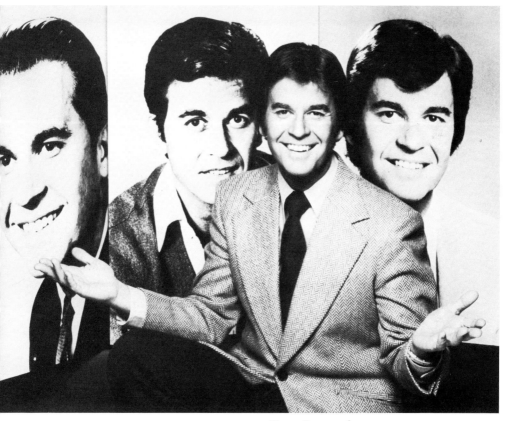

Here I am a few years ago
(note the wide lapels),
standing in front of a photo
montage of Dick Clark in the
'50s, '60s, and '70s. I guess I
haven't changed much.

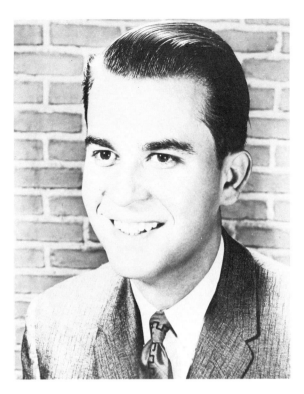

The young Dick Clark, in the late 1950s, shortly after "American Bandstand" went on national television.

Here I am at about age thirty-five in the early to middle 1960s.

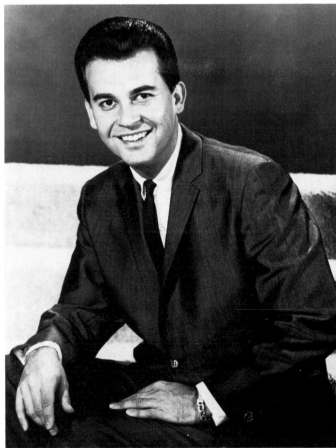

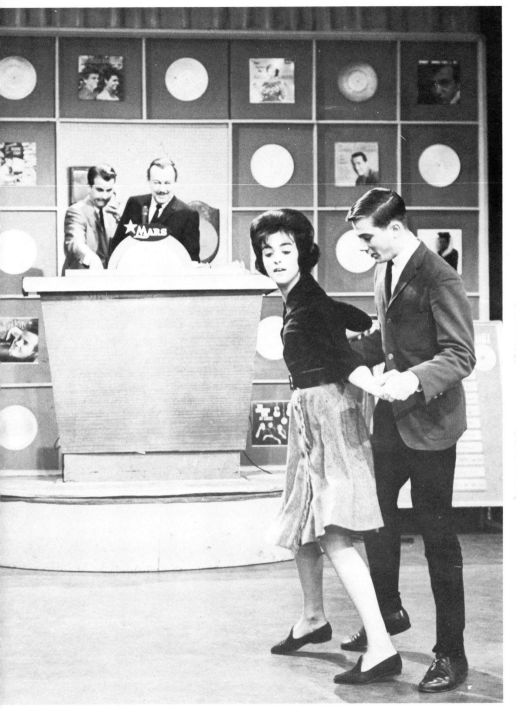

TV quizmaster Jack Barry
and I watch a couple dance
on camera in the middle
1950s.

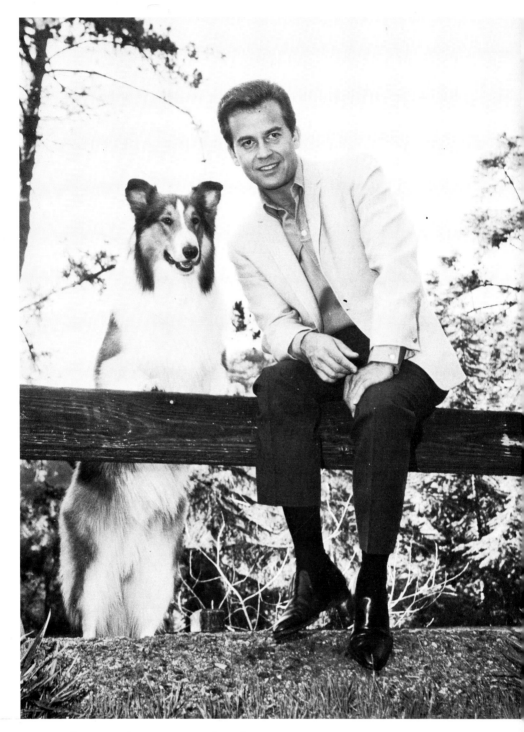

I may not seem to age, but then neither does Lassie — except that they keep replacing the dog. Here I am with Lassie on the dog's show in the 1960s.

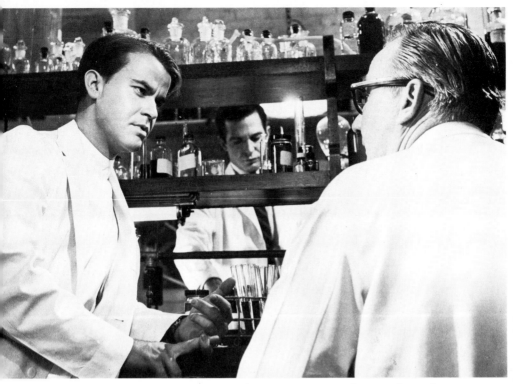

In one of my greatest performances, I confront Edward
Andrews while Ben Gazzara ignores both of us in *The Young
Doctors*, 1961.

We play the music, the kids dance, and I watch during an ABC
"American Bandstand" show in 1966.

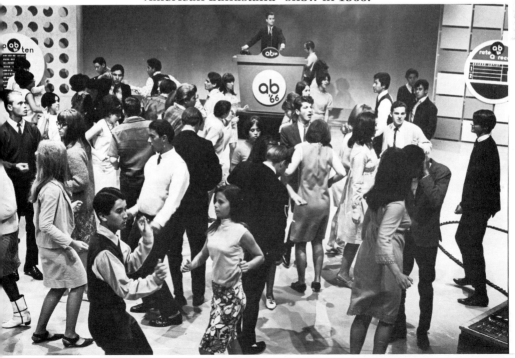

Here, in the 1950s, I talk to a couple of the kids who helped to make the show what it is.

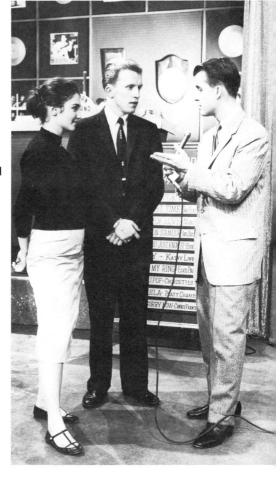

Four of my frequent guests — (from left to right) Paul Anka and Frankie Avalon, front; and Pat Boone and Bobby Darin, back. This was taken after an earlier show — about twenty years ago.

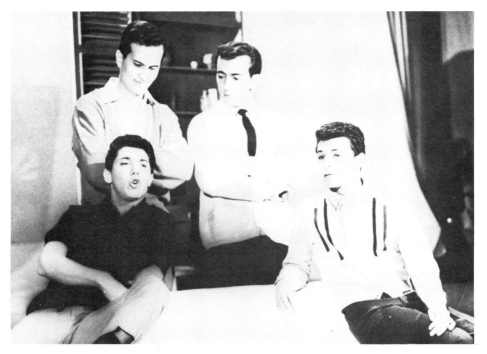

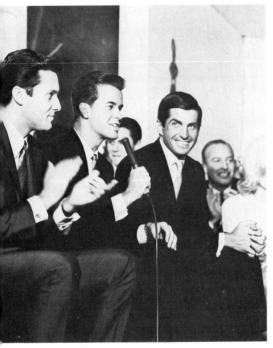

I must have said something so clever that it made Jack Jones, left, applaud and George Hamilton, right, smile. This was in the early 1960s, and I was very clever at that time.

While the group crowds in, I interview Fabian in 1960.

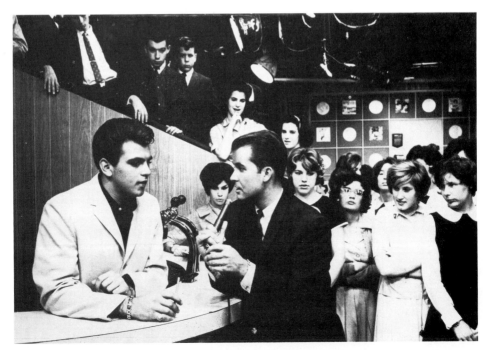

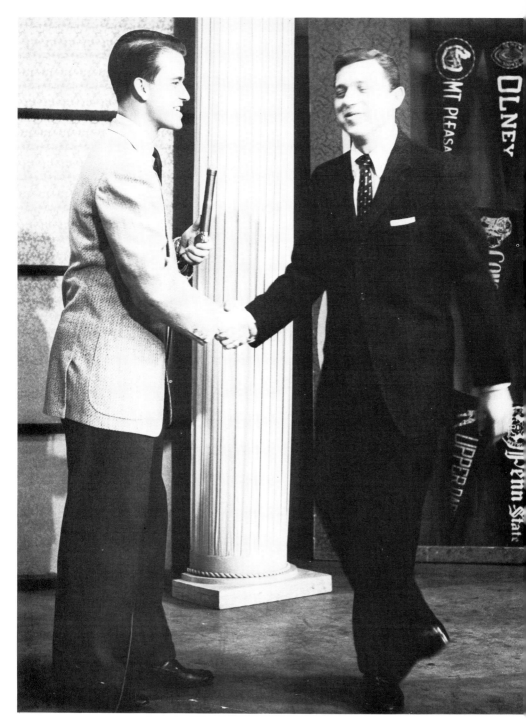

Steve Lawrence is trying to smile, but my handshake in the 1950s was so firm it made him blur with pain.

as many as three hundred people at work at a time, and as few as a couple of dozen. We've had slow times, and I always find it hard to slow down. I remember one time I decided to open a submarine sandwich stand on some property that was available. People said I couldn't do that, that I was in the entertainment business and it would diminish my image to sell subs. I said if other entertainers could open restaurants, I could open a submarine sandwich stand. A lot more people eat subs than steak. As it happens, somebody beat me to it. I was sorry. Still am. The sub business is booming. I think that whatever business I was in, I'd be a compulsive worker.

I like to have a lot of things going on at one time, but I am good at organization. I can dictate a letter to my secretary, talk to a visitor, and make notes on a project at the same time. I have two secretaries, and I keep both of them busy. I apportion projects between them. I have my finger in all the pies, but I am not afraid of delegating authority. I hire the best people I can get, and I let them do their best for me. There are a lot of things a lot of people can do a lot better than I can.

I guess I have a good-sized ego, but it isn't as big as some. For you, one of the keys to getting a lot done in any business is to acknowledge the fact that some people can do some things better than you can and to put these people to work doing these things for you, while you work at doing the things you do best. Many people in authority are unable to delegate authority. They hire people to do things for them, then waste a lot of time looking over the people's shoulders while they try to do these things. They often don't let these people do their work, often wind up doing it for them. They try to carry the load themselves and subject themselves to unnecessary stress and strain. Give yourself a break. Give yourself the benefit of sharing your burdens with others.

If you are organized and plan properly, you can get a lot done without a lot of stress and strain. Do as I do. Make up lists of the things you have to do every day. Put the priority projects on top. If something *has* to be done today, you want to do it ahead of something that can be done tomorrow. Something that has to be done has to be put ahead of something that doesn't have to be done. A lot of the time we do a lot of things that are more interesting but less important than other things. We waste a lot of time on nonsensical things.

At the end of the work day you want to know that you have done the things that should have been done, if not everything you hoped to do. You'll get a sense of satisfaction that will take a lot of tension out of you.

I find that if I concentrate on each thing I have to do in turn, I often can do two days' work in two hours. Concentration is a key. You cannot concentrate by thinking about concentrating. You concentrate by aiming all your attention at each task in turn. Bearing down on the subject of the moment, you concentrate. You have to avoid distractions, clearing your mind of everything that isn't essential to the thing you have to do. You do this by having others screen calls and visitors or by discouraging calls and visitors that do not relate to the thing you are doing at the time you want to do it.

Dr. Marilyn Machlowitz, who has a Ph.D. in management psychology and works for the New York Life Insurance Company, started a study on workaholics for her master's thesis at Yale University in the mid-1970s and since has written extensively on them, interviewing many for a book, *Workaholics.* She has found that workaholics are not all bad, that, in fact, they do things faster and better than the average person does; and I find many of them use my methods. Almost all of them keep lists of things to do, for example. Unfortunately, Dr. Machlowitz found some of them waste a lot of time looking for lost lists, which I find funny.

She is not convinced, as some are, that being a workaholic is unhealthy. She finds that "they get pleasure from working" and says they would be dissatisfied without accomplishments. She does not consider anyone driven by desperation to hard work — such as someone who must pay for a costly sickness in the family or make money to avoid financial failure — to be an authentic workaholic. She considers the true workaholic to be one who works far beyond the norm simply for work's sake and one for whom money or glory is only a measure of success, not success itself.

She would not consider me a true workaholic (though I consider myself one) because I take time out to sleep, eat, go on vacation, and spend time with my family. I do think that if I had taken more time with my family early in my life, I might have had at the least a little better chance of making my first two marriages work. I don't think you should want to be a workaholic to the degree that you risk your marriage and family. Dr. Machlowitz points out that many people she considers to be true workaholics even put the stuff of life on their lists, such as sex with a mate. She says, however, "They tend to put sex down pretty low on their list of priorities." Well, it is not low on my list, and I hope it is not low on your list, and if that makes us less than pure workaholics, so be it. Most of us like to think we work hard, and I'm sure many of you do, but it is the way you work that may make you old before your time.

I think the way for you to avoid excessive stress in your life, while still making the most of your life, is to work hard, devotedly, enthusiastically while you are working, but to take time to rest and to play — and to play hard, devotedly, enthusiastically, while you are playing. Constant exertion or mental tension is exhausting. The mind needs a break.

It will be helpful to you to use your time wisely to clear time for rest and play. Nothing makes you feel worse than wasting time. Nothing is more exhausting than wasted effort. When you procrastinate, when you put off something that has to be done, you feel lousy later. When you get done what had to be done, you feel great afterward. When you just do it, you'll have time left for other things, for a little rest and recreation, for a night out, a weekend off, a vacation.

You have to apportion your time intelligently. You may be able to get a lot done in a little time, but if you allow only one hour to do something that will take you two hours, you're being foolish and are bound to be frustrated. Resisting stress requires, among other things, a realistic look at life.

I have an appearance to make in Virginia. Kari's going with me. We have an apartment in New York we use when we're in the city, and we thought we'd like to stay in it overnight and see some friends. But we have to be back in L.A. the next day. We are trying to figure out how we can leave L.A. in the morning, get to Virginia by noon, make the appearance, fly on to New York, then fly back so we can be in L.A. in time to take care of our business the next day. There are flights we can make, but we realize that if the weather is bad, the flights may be delayed. It scares us just thinking about it. We realize we are imposing artificial stress on ourselves.

We decide to fly to Virginia the night before and spend the night there. We can sleep in, have a leisurely breakfast, and get to my appearance easily. Washington is a lot closer than New York. Kari used to work there and has friends there she's been wanting to see. So we're going to go on to Washington for a while. Then we'll fly back to L.A. and spend the night at our place. I'll be relaxed and refreshed for business in L.A. the next day.

A trip is a trip, but it can be refreshing. Just taking a sensible approach to this trip has relieved me of a lot of anxiety and reduced stress on me. If we had to hustle from here to there in order to meet a strict schedule, we'd have to put a lot of pressure on ourselves.

I think we all have to take holidays, take time off, get away from work in some way. It is, in a way, harder for me, harder for anyone who works for himself than for someone who works for someone else. If you work for yourself, you tend to do more, to stay at it longer. If you get time off as a matter of routine — weekends off and vacations that are scheduled — you take off. In any event, I believe it is important to get away, so I do.

Kari and I take a lot of short trips. I'd rather take a lot of short breaks than one long vacation. It spaces the year out better. We try to go places we haven't been, new places that will be different from what we know, where we can lead a life different from the life we usually lead. We look forward to each vacation with youthful anticipation, and I think it keeps us young.

Some people stop taking trips. They've been here and they've been there. They feel they can't take the time. They get out of the habit. For us, a night in the mountains, two days in Las Vegas, or a weekend in Santa Barbara is super. And if we can go somewhere we haven't been, that's better yet. For you, a good short trip may be anywhere in your area, for there is no area that doesn't have something interesting to attract a visit. There is no area that doesn't have something interesting no farther away than a comfortable car ride.

The area expands into other interesting places if you take a train ride or bus tour. The airlines frequently offer special low fares for certain trips. A cruise, as I mentioned earlier, may be within reach. As I suggested, check with a travel agent. When you get back to business after one of these relaxers, you'll feel refreshed and ready to roll again.

It is a fact that the highest homicide rate in this country comes on Saturdays, the highest suicide rate on Mondays. I figure people are so tense from their work week that by the weekend they're ready to explode. If the weekend hasn't repaired the damage that has been done, the dread of returning to the old routine makes them suicidal. They just can't face another week. If the pressures of your work are too much for you, get into some other work. It's that simple. You may feel you can't afford to do it. It may be that you can't afford not to do it.

Statistics show that midweek is the safest time. For most of us the routine is restful, comfortable. We can work at keeping it this way, I believe, with coffee breaks. They give the mind and muscles time to rest and regenerate their vigor so that we can return to work refreshed. Stop-and-go sports are like this. The pause between pitches and plays gives ballplayers time for their strength to return. Running is rougher because you have to keep going. They say real wrestling, as the amateurs do it, is the most exhausting because in certain holds the muscles are at tension for prolonged periods and do not get time to restore their strength and energy.

You have to relax to recharge your mental batteries, too. Too rigid a routine is not restful; it increases stress. If you have breakfast at seven, lunch at twelve, and dinner at six every day of your life, if you have toast and coffee every morning, it throws you out of whack on days you can't stick to the schedule. If you have to do a certain thing at one o'clock every afternoon and have to go to bed at eleven every night, it poses a real problem when you can't.

Variety is the spice of life. I have my routine, but part of my routine is to alter the routine as life dictates. The body tells us a lot if we'll listen. Every day is different. The demands of every day are different. Whenever possible and within reason, if I feel tired, I lie down. If I feel hungry, I eat. If I'm not tired, I keep going. If I'm not hungry, I skip a meal. Some days I require more rest than others. Some mornings I go for a big breakfast. You should alter your routine to your mood.

I tend to start late and finish late, go to bed late and get up late. But I'm not a robot, and I don't think anyone should live life automatically. If you get used to change, change won't affect you. Taking a two- or three-hour plane ride upsets some businessmen. To me it's the same as sitting down to a two- or three-hour meal with someone. Some people are affected by the so-called jet lag as they travel. I'm a coast-to-coast character, and I don't suffer from jet lag. I think a lot of this stuff is in the mind. I don't think about these things. I work as long as I have to. When I'm tired, I sleep. When I'm hungry, I eat. Try it.

Locking yourself into rigid routines that do not allow for variety will make you old before your time. Varying your routine is the youthful thing. Doing things on the spur of the moment refreshes you. In a way you look forward to each day a lot more if you don't know what each day will bring. Don't pass up a chance to do something you'd like to do that suddenly turns up just because you hadn't planned to do it.

Don't rush through lunch. Allow time for it. This is your midday break, and it's critical to your composure. Taking time for it, you'll find you can make more of the rest of your time. Most of us are surrounded by co-workers most of the time. If at all possible, try to be by yourself part of the time.

Meditation is marvelous, for the time you keep for yourself. A few moments of meditation can work wonders. In Transcendental Meditation you are asked to get into a comfortable position in a quiet place and repeat one word over and over — a word like "love" or "peace" or "happiness" — while otherwise making your mind as blank as possible. TM therapists recommend twenty minutes of this in the morning and again in the evening. Some therapists recommend a lot of exotic trappings. At least I think they are trappings; I don't think they are necessary.

You may not have a lot of time, but I do think it is important to take some time to sit quietly and try to free your mind of your problems. If you can do it in nature, surrounded by beauty, it can be enormously relaxing. It can reduce stress.

Make sure you get all the rest you need. I try to get eight hours' sleep a night, but often can't. I take naps to make up for it. Naps are my secret remedy. While our home is in Malibu, we have a living area, including a bedroom, in the building that serves as our Hollywood office. Sometimes, when my schedule is tight, Kari and I sleep over at the office. And I can take naps there in one of my own beds, instead of crunching up on a couch. Maybe even a couch is out of the question for you, but perhaps you can work something out that will permit a comfortable nap.

We sleep on firm, almost hard mattresses and firm, almost hard pillows. We often take some of the stuffing out of a new pillow. I believe firmness is best for the body in general, and for the back in particular for rest and posture. We sleep on satin sheets and pillowcases. It sounds like a luxury, but they're not that expensive. And they're comfortable and kind to the skin. Beauty experts swear by satin pillows. I just happen to like them, and the side benefit of their being good to your complexion is a bonus.

Eight hours' sleep a night is traditional. And I find it really works best for me. A different amount may work best for you. You know how much sleep you need. You know how too much or too little sleep affects you. For instance, I find I can do fine with seven hours, but I can't function well with six. Too little sleep leaves me limp, just as too much makes me logy. I can't always work enough sleep time into my schedule. I may be up late and have to get up early. For me, naps supply the solution. You have to find your sleep solution, too. But find one. You can't work well, play well, or do anything well when you're tired.

Naps worked for Thomas Edison. He got by with four hours a night because he took four or five short naps a day. Some as brief as ten or fifteen minutes. If you actually fall asleep, even a one-minute nap works. Sometimes you drift off for a few seconds, wake up, and are surprised at how little time has elapsed yet how refreshed you feel. Some people complain that they feel worse when they wake up from a nap than they did when they lay down, but I think you will find that if you return to work slowly, you soon will feel better and will be refreshed and have renewed energy.

Edison used to drift off in the middle of meetings or boring conversations. Maybe he could get away with this. Most of us can't, even if we'd like to. Most of us have to find a place where we can be alone and not be accused of sleeping on the job. Unfortunately, some of us can't do this.

Something that works for those who can get in a short nap is a slant board. All day we are standing or sitting. The blood drains to our feet. A slant board lets you lie with your feet up and your head down. It allows the blood to flow back through your body and into your brain. Five minutes on a slant board is remarkably refreshing. It is astonishing how well your thinking process improves.

Some of us are so busy trying to do things that we don't take the time to think them through so that we can do them as well, as swiftly, and as efficiently as they can be done. Prepared properly, we work faster and better.

One thing that works well for me is deep breathing. Some of us are so busy that we don't even take the time to breathe right. We get going, and we get into shallow breathing. But our bodies need oxygen. Tests show that in meditation the heart rate slows down, breathing becomes shallow, and we need less oxygen. But the more active we are, the faster our heartbeat, the greater demand our body has for oxygen.

Try this: Breathe deeply through your nose into your stomach, hold it a second, then slowly let the air come up, exhaling through your mouth. This kind of breathing is a form of yoga and it works. A lot of yoga works. Take the time to breathe deeply periodically, and your body will benefit.

My dentist told me the other day that my gums looked bad, so business must be bad. He was partly right. Business isn't bad, but it had been a bad day. I was surprised it showed in my gums. The degree of stress we are experiencing is sometimes reflected in our appearance. Sometimes I start to see lines on my forehead, dark rings under my eyes, and redness in my eyes. When I see these danger signs, I slow down and take a break. If I feel tired, I rest. The rigors of the road, of cross-country tours, sometimes have made me tired to the bone. I suspect this is dangerous. It certainly can age you.

A feeling of fatigue, sore muscles, an aching back, a lack of wind, and a loss of appetite all are signs of stress. The blood pressure rises, the heartbeat increases, the lungs dilate. We do not get the blood and oxygen through our bodies that we need. You don't have to be a doctor to understand this. One doctor, William Klein, a Westminster, California, internist, says, "The links from overwork and exhaustion to heart trouble, strokes, hypertension, and the like are clear, though other things cause these, too. The chemistry of the body dictates how well we can stand up to stress and sickness, but the overworked, exhausted body is less resistant to physical problems. You have to work efficiently and take time off for repairs if you are going to work well or even go on working."

A person who is tired is old. He looks tired, he looks old. I believe we can handle a lot of work, and work well, look young and feel young, if we organize our schedules intelligently, if we prepare properly, if we put the most effort to the priority items, if we take time off, if we use our time wisely, if we rest properly and eat right, and if we clear our minds so that we can think straight. I believe we can resist stress, and thus resist aging and illness, if we think our lives through and do those things that are smart to do. If we know we are right about the way we are living our lives, we will feel better about our lives and ourselves.

I think the only way you will feel good and look good is to look at yourself and feel good about yourself.

4
Looking Good

What makes us look good? Good looks, of course. But we're either born with good looks or we're not. We can, however, make the most of our looks. There are things we can do to make ourselves look good.

Let's look at what makes us look bad, aside from the fates. Poor health. Too much weight. Bad posture. Bad skin and bad teeth. Messy hair and clothes.

What makes us look old? Gray hair or loss of hair. Loss of teeth. Wrinkled, sagging skin or sagging flesh. A slowed-down step. Out-of-date hairstyles and clothes.

One of the experts to whom I went for advice said that the three factors that most make someone look old are excess weight, poor posture, and deliberate movements. The expert pointed out that people of any age may be fat, but that to look slim is to look youthful. And he added that agile, confident movement definitely looks youthful.

Another expert classified personality and appearance types by seasons and said I was a "spring," as opposed to, say, a "fall." This one said of me, "Dick is an ingenue, and ingenues never really age. He is slender, compact, and has good posture. He wears his hair in good style and dresses fashionably. He always appears neat. He is clear-eyed and appears healthy and agile. He has that blondish coloring that wears gracefully and a youthful personality that wears well."

Very nice. Ingenue, eh? Again, a lot of it is luck. I was born with my coloring, and I've been blessed with good health. I've been blessed with good eyes and good teeth and a full head of hair.

But I've had to work to keep my weight down and my posture up. I take care of my body and my teeth and my skin. I take care of my hair and my clothes, and I'm conscious of fashion.

I'm getting a few gray hairs. Personally, I think a little gray looks good. On some people, even a lot looks good. I haven't dyed my hair, but if I get a lot of gray and I think it ages me — if I don't think it looks good — I'll get it dyed in a minute and not feel the slightest embarrassment about it.

I do and I will continue to do whatever I can do to keep my youthful appearance. Looking around, I'd say the average person could look a lot younger and a lot better if he worked at it just a little.

Looking young doesn't mean looking good. But looking good does mean, at least in part, looking young.

Being young certainly doesn't guarantee good looks. A person in his teens or twenties who is sloppy doesn't look good, even to other young people.

Traditionally, teen-agers suffer from acne. Many have crooked teeth. With parental help, doctors and dentists can do a lot to correct these problems. If it isn't done then, a person in his twenties, as he moves out on his own, or even someone in this thirties, forties, and fifties, can take care of these things. It's never too late.

You're never too old to improve your appearance. And the result of many of these improvements will be to make you look younger as well as make you better-looking. It is easy to do many of these things. Most of them should come naturally. Cleanliness, for example.

Wash your hands and face thoroughly several times a day. A thousand things soil our skin during the day. Even the air is no longer clean. Look at the dust and dirt that accumulates on outdoor furniture. It accumulates on you, too. And keep your fingernails trim and clean. Nothing looks worse than dirty fingernails.

Do I sound like a parent talking to a child? Perhaps, but sometimes we have to talk to ourselves as if we were children. Sometimes when we get busy we get out of the good habits many of us learned, and we all should have learned, as children.

If you have a mate or a lover, get her to look out for you. And you look out for her. If you're personal with someone, be personal. If you care for someone, care — and let that someone care for you. We don't see ourselves as others see us. Don't be afraid to ask about yourself. And encourage those close to you to take advice. Don't be unkind, but be kind.

We should want to know if we have food on our lips or in our teeth, caught in a mustache or beard. We should want to know if the back of our neck or ears or the backs of our arms or our elbows are dirty. We should want to know if we have bad breath or body odor.

Brush your teeth thoroughly and use a mouthwash several times a day if possible. Use breath mints if necessary.

Shower every day before you go out for
the day, and, if necessary, again before
you go out for the evening. Wash as well
as you can the back of your neck and
behind your ears, places that so often
and in so many ways get soiled. Wash the
backs of your arms and elbows. Use a
deodorant and talcum powder after
every shower.

A dip in the pool or ocean or lake
isn't a shower. You get wet and you get
the dust off, but you don't get clean. A
bath is nice, but it is not a substitute for
a shower, and it isn't for cleanliness. You
can't soap up and rinse off and sit in a
tubful of dirty, soapy water and get clean.

A bath is a bath is a bath. A hot tub is
very restful. It softens the skin and re-
laxes the muscles. It eases sore weari-
ness.

Actually lukewarm water is better for
the skin than hot water is. Adding a little
baby oil to the water helps soften the
skin. Or you can add a little milk, even
powdered milk. It's no old-wives' tale.
Beauticians say a pint of milk added to
bath water is beneficial to the skin. I prefer a bath gel, which removes dead skin
and scales. It feels and smells good.

Don't take a lot of baths, but if you
like them, they may be helpful to you
and to your skin in different ways. It may
be restful for you, and it will lubricate
and soften your skin.

The ladies usually add some cologne

after they come out of the shower or
bath and dry off. Men can add a little,
too, or talc. It seems to stick better when
the skin is warm and the pores are still
open. Not too much. You don't want a
noticeable smell. Like the ladies, men
can put a little oil into their skin. Baby oil
is fine, by the way.

Use a deodorant, of course. You don't
want a bad smell. In my youth, the
commercials called it B.O. — body odor.
That was telling it like it was. And is. We
all know some people who, to put it
bluntly, smell bad. You don't want to get
close to them. Don't take a chance of
being one of them. Shower.

I suggest using a body moisturizer af-
terwards. It helps restore the skin's natural softness and helps to prevent dry-
ness.

When I was young, I had oily skin
and the traditional acne. The acne was a
big pain.

Like most youngsters, I hated it. Time
took care of it for me. It doesn't for
everyone. Your face will look bad if you
have acne. And it's a serious psychological problem for anyone who has it.

Dermatologists can do wonders today
with all kinds of acne. Many drugstore
lotions won't do what the ads say they
will, though some do help. A good der-
matologist can not only treat you effectively but can steer you to effective home
care of acne. It's worth the cost.

Soap and water remains the basic treatment for acne, but special lotions will help. Facials given by specialists cleanse the skin. Women get facials regularly, but most men are too embarrassed. Why? Shouldn't a man care about his appearance? Isn't your skin a critical part of your appearance? You may want to try a home treatment — one of the men's face masks. They're easy to apply in privacy. More and more men aren't shy about using them.

We men have to get over our self-consciousness if we are going to make a real effort to look good. I use skin creams. There, one of my secrets is out. I don't think of myself as *macho*, but I sure don't think using skin cream makes me less *macho*.

As I got older, my oily skin began to dry out. Whether this came from age or from the makeup television performers use regularly or from some other factor, my skin began to feel rough and brittle, and I wasn't too happy about it.

One night as I lay in bed watching my lady clean up, getting ready to go to sleep, I noticed that she applied skin cream to her face. I thought, "Why shouldn't I?" Why shouldn't a man? I asked her about it. She said, "Why not?"

I've used skin cream every night since. Actually, I use a moisturizer. I've experimented with several to try to find a combination I like. I finally concocted a formula that works for me. This is one of several products I've designed. I put the name Dick Clark on them because I've experimented on them for years, finding my own way to fight the ravages of time. I find it keeps my skin soft and contributes considerably to a youthful appearance.

Nothing is going to make me as good-looking as Robert Redford, but maybe I can look a little younger.

Dry skin is thin and has small pores, so it seldom has pimples, but it is sensitive and tends to blemishes and flakiness. Oily skin is thicker, has larger and more visible pores, is less sensitive and flaky, but is more prone to pimples. My oily skin proved a blessing to me as I got older, because everyone's skin tends to dry out as he gets older. Most people have in-between skin to begin with, neither excessively oily or dry, but any skin requires care.

Every morning you have to clean not only your face but also your chin and neck. I find it better to use a moisturizing cleansing bar. Soap may tend to dry out your skin. Once a week, use a deep-cleansing lotion to clear out your pores. Then apply an astringent. Whatever your skin type, it takes only a few seconds to apply a moisturizer and a few minutes to let it work for you. It's worth the time. For obvious reasons I recommend my own Dick Clark brand for morning use. It contains PABA, a clinically proven sun-screening element. It filters out the damaging sun rays that contribute to wrinkles, lines, and premature aging of your skin.

Rub a moisturizer deep into your skin from your neck to your hairline. Use some on your hands, elbows, and even your feet if the skin seems dry. Many people apply moisturizers abundantly, but it shouldn't show. Use only a little bit, but rub it in good. You don't have to buy the most expensive kind. In moisturizers, the extra cost comes from extra perfume. And perfume is perfume is perfume.

Moisturizers really are a skin coating. They keep the skin's natural moisture in and the drying and dirtying elements of the outside world out. If you have oily skin, you do not need as much as if you have dry skin. You need less in the summer, more in the winter. But a good moisturizer will help protect you from the sun.

Many people are sun worshippers. They seek suntans. On many people a suntan looks super. But science has learned that too much sun dries out your skin too much and may even contribute to skin cancer. So, be careful. Know the risks before you lie in the sun too long.

If you have sensitive skin, blemishes, eczema, or some other skin problem, you probably will benefit from hypoallergenic soaps or lotions. These do not contain the irritating chemicals and perfumes that otherwise may make the soap and lotion attractive to you. Many women wear hypoallergenic makeup.

Hypoallergenic products are not totally irritant free, however. And they do not last too long because they do not contain chemical preservatives, so buy them in small amounts and replace them regularly. The beautiful ladies in my business tell me they buy all their cosmetics in small amounts and replace them regularly to make sure what they use is fresh.

Personally, I like the looks of a lady with either very little makeup or makeup that does not show. I'll never know why anyone thinks she looks good with a lot of makeup on, though some exotic beauties can get away with it. If women never wore makeup, as most men do not, the sexes would be equal!

Actually, my hairstylist tells me an increasing number of men are starting to wear makeup, feeling they can cover up that haggard look that may come from a hard day's work before they go out at night. He says this makeup consists primarily of shadowing and highlighting, perhaps some eyebrow or eyelash work, and that it doesn't show. I'm not so sure it wouldn't.

I wear makeup on camera so I know

that beauty experts can work wonders with makeup, but I don't need much and I don't think I could get away with it off camera and away from the artificial lighting. I wouldn't even want to try. And I don't think you can conceal wrinkles with makeup. I think the older ladies who lay it on heavily in the hopes of doing this only accentuate their age. I do think that a wise woman could do worse than to ask a beautician how to apply makeup because the best beauticians paint faces with the skill of an artist painting a canvas.

One of the best things a fellow can do after a hard day and before a night out is to take a shower to freshen up. Another thing that really refreshes you and your appearance is a fresh shave. Be sure to use a shaving cream that contains a good moisturizer. I also use an after-shave moisturizer rather than an alcohol-based lotion. A moisturizer gives you the same refreshing feeling that doesn't dry out your skin.

Of course, the way we men shave is about as barbaric as the way some women paint their faces. When you think about it, scraping the hair off your face with sharp metal is strange. Clearly, it's not natural.

Yet I don't like to see a woman with hair on her legs or under her arms, and I think they should remove such body hair.

Savages didn't shave. Safety razors and double-edge blades came after the cavemen. Certainly electric razors did. But these are modern times, and I personally prefer a clean-shaven look. I am light-haired and do not have an exceptionally heavy beard. I use a blade. Many light-bearded men prefer the convenience of an electric razor. The darker and heavier your beard, the more you will need the closer cut of a razor blade.

One beauty expert points out that you could throw a light-haired, light-skinned type like Robert Redford in the woods for a week without a shave and he'd come out looking great, but you could leave an equally good-looking but dark-skinned, dark-haired type like Robert Goulet in the woods for a week without a shave and he'd come out looking like a bum.

Although they're not for me, mustaches and beards are in style now. They are readily accepted. Some men look good in mustaches and beards, some do not. A lot depends on how a man looks to himself in a mustache or beard. In some cases a beard can conceal a fault in your facial structure, such as a weak chin or a jutting jaw.

A mustache does not always make a man look older. And in some cases it may take the eye away from a nose that may be too large or lips that may be too full.

Burt Reynolds is an example of a prominent man who sometimes wears a mustache and sometimes doesn't, and I think it is difficult to decide if he looks better or older with or without one. I guess Burt would look good in any case.

A mustache will make most men look older. A beard will definitely do so. Of course, some young men with youthful faces may want to look older. I should have worn a beard back in the days when I was removed from doing the news and those beer commercials on television because I looked too young. Now, when I start to grow a bit of a beard just for the fun of it, like when I'm away on a vacation, I find a lot of gray growing in it, and I shave it off fast.

If, for whatever reason, you want to wear a mustache or beard, keep it neatly trimmed and at an appropriate length. What is an appropriate length? It depends on the shape of your face. See your barber or hairstylist for expert advice, just as you should when deciding about the length of your hair. Again, neatness is a key to keeping a good, youthful appearance. A fashionable cut and length is another key to this.

The length of your hair is no tip-off to your age. Many young men wear their hair longer than their girl friends do. But the older fellow who wears his hair real long does not usually look younger for it. A younger man is better able to get away with shaggy, unkempt hair, especially if he is wearing jeans or shorts or a bathing suit, but no one is going to look good this way.

Long hair was in for a long time, but I guess it's going out today. I don't think we'll go back to crewcuts or the short look of the 1940s, but we seem to be getting away from the long look of the '70s. I'm seeing ears and the backs of necks again. In any event, it is important to a youthful look to keep up with the styles and be in fashion. Look around you or at fashionable magazines, or ask your barber or hairstylist to keep up with the trends.

I don't want to put barbers out of business, but I believe the biggest advance in the appearance of men in my time has been the practice of hairstyling for men. I think all men should have their hair styled and not merely cut. A hairstylist charges more, but it's usually worth it. A hairstylist shapes your hair to the shape of your head and cuts it so that your hair will keep its shape without being brushed or combed or oiled down extensively. Of course, many barbers are trained as stylists, too. You want to go to someone who is trained and can do your hair in a way that makes you happy.

Myself, I go to a beauty salon that has as many men customers as women and works on both equally well. There are some big names among the men, but I won't give their names because they might be embarrassed by it, though I don't think they should be. Many men not only get their hair styled but get it permed, dyed, and so forth. Many get facials and manicures. Why not? Why shouldn't a man care as much about his appearance as a woman does? Your appearance is no measure of your real masculinity.

If a man is going to keep his hair neat and in fashion, he should go to a stylist about once every two weeks and take care of his hair in between visits. With a good styling, you won't look like you just stepped out of the chair. You need to get a lot chopped off only if you go to the stylist only every month or two. You should find a stylist you like and go to the same one all the time to keep a consistency to your cut. When I'm out of town and can't get to my regular stylist, I go to a stylist and ask him to trim my hair along the lines set by my regular stylist. I have yet to find a hairstylist who is offended by this. A stylist can appreciate consistency and loyalty as much as anyone.

I shampoo my hair regularly, at least daily, always in a lukewarm shower because I can rinse out the shampoo best in a shower. I am told by experts that the old belief that too much shampoo robs your hair of its natural oils is not true, especially with the new, milder shampoos available today. You can shampoo every day in every shower if you want, and you can shampoo twice at a time to make sure you are getting your hair clean. It is important to rinse out the shampoo thoroughly. I shampoo in lukewarm, soft water. And I am careful to rinse out the shampoo thoroughly.

I blot the excess water off my hair, then let it dry naturally. I use a hand-held dryer if necessary and portion my hair with a wide-toothed comb while I am using a dryer. I use a soft brush to help my hair into its styled place. Many men don't use a dryer. It's not necessary if your hair has been styled properly, for your hair usually will fall into its proper place naturally. But if you use a dryer, you have to use it properly. You have to keep it at least half an arm's length away from your hair and keep it moving to keep it from burning or singeing your hair.

I use very little hair spray because I like a natural, slightly windblown look to my hair, and I don't like the scents of most sprays. Fewer men are using hair spray now than did a few years ago because the natural, slightly windblown look is in. However, "grease" seems to be coming back in, and a lot of fellows are applying a little oil, especially to the sides of their hair, to give their hair a shine. I'm not.

There are conditioners that add body

to your hair and highlight your natural
hair color; rinses that penetrate your hair
and color it until it gradually washes out
with each shampooing; and dyes and
bleaches that, though not permanent, do
not wash out for a long time. I haven't
yet felt the need to dye my hair in any
way, though I would if I did.

More women dye their hair than
men, though more men are doing it
every year. Society seems to accept gray
hair on a man more than it does on a
woman. In some cases, gray, especially in
the sideburns and at the temples, seems
to make a man look distinguished. If you
like gray, fine. But I do think gray ages a
man as much as it does a woman.

Ronald Reagan swears he doesn't dye
his hair, that he simply hasn't gone gray,
not even in the sideburns where gray
usually begins. Eager-beaver reporters
have searched his barber shop for clip-
pings that would reveal that he dyes, but
have been unable to produce any proof.
So I assume he is telling the truth. But at
his age his hair doesn't look natural, so
maybe he'd actually be better off coloring
his sideburns gray to keep rumors away.

Johnny Carson admits he used to dye
his hair. He wanted to continue looking
young on his "Tonight" show. Then he
decided he'd feel better about himself
with the natural color of his hair. He let it
grow out to its natural color, and now it
is completely gray. He looks older, but he

doesn't look *old*. He looks good and feels good about it. It's up to the individual.

Few men can get away with changing their hair color the way women do. What society accepts in a woman, in this case, it simply has not yet come around to accept in a man. Any man who suddenly changes from black hair to blond is going to startle those he deals with every day and will probably look foolish, not younger.

As for the ladies, I don't believe blonds have more fun, but if you do, become a blond. If you're a blond and feel you'll look better as a brunette, be a brunette. But do ask the advice of your friends and loved ones, and your beautician or hairstylist.

Change is not always for the better. Once, years ago, Connie Francis came on my show with her black hair dyed deep red. I was so startled I asked her what the heck she'd done to herself before I bit my tongue. She was as hurt as my tongue was. But after she got more than a thousand letters the next few days telling her the public liked her better the way they knew her, with black hair, she removed the red.

It is not always easy to remove the red or other coloring, and it is easy to come out of a coloring session with pretty strange coloring. It also is easy to do damage to your hair during a coloring session. So, while some products in the stores are good products, I think you would be wise to have an expert apply any coloring you may want.

Similarly, I think you would be wise to have an expert pick out a wig or hairpiece for you and fit it to you. Women wear different-colored, different-styled wigs from day to day, night to night; men don't, but more and more men are wearing toupees of some kind these days. I don't because I don't need one; but if I did, I would.

Men wearing hairpieces has been a commonplace in show business for many years. They get good ones that don't show. A lot of people say they can always tell when someone is wearing a hairpiece, but the truth is many men are wearing good ones that no one notices. If you want a hairpiece, get a good one.

Among many others, Frank Sinatra wears a hairpiece. Sometimes Burt Reynolds uses a piece to fill in. I don't think they show. Many stars don't care if anyone knows. Carl Reiner goes on television without his hairpiece as often as he does with it. His son, Rob, also wears one. You don't have to be a glamour guy going bald to want to maintain a good head of hair. But only a specialist can fit a good hairpiece to you properly.

Many men don't really notice when they are beginning to lose their hair. Often, the loss begins in a small area at the upper back of the head, and you can't see the bald spot unless you look in a double mirror. Frequently, a helpful friend will tell you. Perhaps the thinning hair won't bother you. But if it does, do something about it.

I've known a lot of men who've looked foolish by trying to comb a few hairs over a bald spot in an attempt to conceal it. I've also known a lot of men who've looked foolish with hair weaves that didn't work well and a few who've suffered damage to their scalps with improper implants. I really recommend you consult someone who knows what he's doing.

I have consulted with a couple of experts for you — Kenneth Craig of the Silvio Pensanti Salon in Studio City, California, who styles my hair, and Jean Donielle of the John LaJoie Salon of Beverly Hills — and I'll let them give you some tips about what's in and what's out and what to do with hairstyles, hair care, hairpieces, mustaches and beards.

As for mustaches and beards, Kenneth says, "They tend to add age and make a man look more mature, which may or may not be good, but some men do look good in them or feel good about themselves in them. More men can wear mustaches effectively than can wear beards. Beards definitely add years to a man, but they can partially conceal a face a man may not like. A mustache can take the eyes away from a nose that is too large or not well-shaped. A beard can conceal a weak chin or a strong chin. An angular beard angled down from the cheekbones can cut down the roundness of a face that may be too round, and a full, round beard can add fullness to an angular, narrow face. Both can cover up double chins. Real thick mustaches are not in, but the trend is toward fairly full mustaches.

"Personally, I don't like mustaches that hang down over the lips, or beards that grow on the lips. These tend to catch particles of food a person is eating, and few things look less attractive.

"A man would be wise to consult his stylist about the size and shape of his mustache or beard and have the stylist trim it properly, then follow these lines while maintaining a mustache or beard at home. He is going to have to have a program of home maintenance because face hair grows fast and will require daily care between visits to a stylist. A small pair of manicure scissors will give a person a delicate touch for trimming a mustache or beard. A razor has to be used carefully. Even if a man does not shave with an electric razor, he might want to buy one that has one of those pop-up trimmers because these work well in trimming mustaches and beards."

Jean adds, "Many men do not realize that you have to brush a beard or mustache just the way you do your hair if you are going to train it to fall into place properly. While mustaches and beards are not to my taste, they are popular and they will look fine if they are fashioned to fit your face and if they are kept trim and neat. Many men decide they want a certain type of mustache or beard without taking a long look at the type of face they have and without thinking about what they want a mustache or beard to do for them. Many men need expert advice, but they don't seek it out. They may think a mustache is distinguished, for example, or a beard manly, and that they can let them go shaggy, but if they care about their appearance they will fashion mustaches and beards properly and care for their facial hair."

As for the length of the hair on our heads, Jean notes, "The trend is toward shorter hair, not quite the Ivy League look, but the style doesn't look like you just stepped out of the chair, and it's not as structured as it was in recent years. I don't believe we will go all the way back to the short look of years ago, but I think we will stay with the ears and neck exposed for some time to come. A good styling will cost $25 to $30, but it will be worth it."

Kenneth leans to a little longer hair: "Right now I like hair that covers the upper part of the ear and drops to the collar, but not to the shoulder. But a man can go a little longer or a little shorter without going out of fashion. Real long hair is out, and I think the medium length is very practical for most purposes."

The expert from Silvio Pensanti's adds, "We now are into casual, soft styles that look natural, rather than the hard, set styles that were popular for a while. Fewer men are using hair spray to fix their hair, though there is a return to oils and gels to slick the sides back a bit. The wet look is definitely in.

"Blow dryers still are in, but a lot of dryers the public can buy provide too much heat and not enough blowing power. You should hold your hair dryer at least six inches away and never concentrate it on one area at a time. Ideally, you should comb out your hair after washing it, go somewhere and do something while it dries, then blow it into place while running your fingers through it to get it right. I prefer combing to brushing."

The expert from John LaJoie's says, "I prefer brushes to combs, but it really doesn't matter because if your hair has been styled properly, it will fall into place properly without either. If your hair has been styled properly, you can dry it while driving with the window open and air blowing on it and it will fall into place, especially with today's casual look.

"Some say use a circular motion with a hair dryer, but I am one who prefers a back-and-forth motion. It really doesn't matter as long as you keep it moving and far enough away not to singe the hair. A good rule of thumb is, if you can feel the heat on your scalp, you are too close."

Jean says, "A man should keep his hair clean and he can shampoo it as often as he wants, every day if he feels it is necessary, as long as he uses a mild shampoo, which has a low pH level. If the label on his shampoo doesn't show this level, which runs from one to ten, or if it shows it and it isn't seven or less, preferably around four or five, then the chances are it is too high and he should seek another shampoo or the advice on a shampoo from his stylist. The advice might be more sincere if the stylist doesn't, himself, sell shampoo."

Kenneth adds, "The pH factor is the acidity factor and it is only overly acidic shampoos that rob the hair of its natural oils. At a level of five pH or so, I recommend a man shower and shampoo every day. Rinse your hair out before shampooing so that the shampoo doesn't have to work too hard. Blot your hair with a dry, soft towel after shampooing and rinsing to remove the excess moisture, letting your hair dry as naturally as possible."

As for hair coloring, Kenneth says, "Most men color their hair to remove or reduce gray, though many come into our salon for highlighting and a few for a totally different color. I feel strongly that anything you do should be done for you by a stylist. This is true for women, too. Most people know they have brown hair or blond hair or whatever, but they don't know the exact shade they have. There are countless shades of each color, and the dying process must match the proper color precisely. Also, as you dye your hair, the color changes, and each succeeding time you dye it, you have to use a slightly different shade. And there are some well-advertised dyes available in stores that will turn gray hair green, for example, and literally harm your hair."

Jean says, "It is not so much that the products on the shelves of stores are bad, but that the directions are often not good, and few can follow the directions right. There is not a large factor in getting the precise color into your hair you want, and if you are doing it for yourself or a friend is doing it for you, you are not apt to be precise. It takes training and extensive experience to apply coloring correctly, and, frankly, I feel your hair is worth this kind of care."

As for hairpieces, he says, "I think they're fine, but they have to be of good quality and fine fit. When someone who is going bald asks me to cut his hair long on one side so he can circle it around and try to cover up a bare spot, I won't do it because I think this only calls attention to the spot. I'd rather recommend a place where he can purchase a quality piece that is matched to his hair color with all a color's variations. Then he can bring the hairpiece to me to cut into place, although this is touchy because if I cut too much in any area of a hairpiece, it's not going to grow back.

"There are some excellent hairpieces available, and the really good ones do run $600 or more, although price is not the only criterion to apply. It has to feel like your hair and look like your hair. The size of your bald area does not matter because all the pieces are put together full and are cut down to the proper shape. This cutting is critical because your hair is not the same thickness and length all around your head, and a piece has to be cut to conform to these variations as well as colored to conform to your varied color if it is not going to be noticeable.

"A good hair weave costs about $5,000, but there have been some good results with these. New hair matching your hair coloring is tied in small knots to existing hair, filling out your head of hair. You can shower and swim freely, as you can with many of today's hairpieces. You do have to return every three weeks or so to have the knots lowered and re-tightened on a hair weave, however, but you also have to have your remaining hair styled more often than usual if you are wearing a hairpiece so it remains the right length for the hairpiece.

"I am not keen on implants because I believe they are too costly for their prospects of success and too dangerous. In these implants, doctors put plugs of synthetic hair into the scalp and tie these in knots beneath the scalp. The scalp frequently rejects them. I've known clients to spend $15,000 to have this done; it took many visits, they suffered much discomfort, and they wound up losing all the hair in six weeks and, in some cases, suffering infection."

Kenneth concludes, "I don't like the look of hair weaves and, while I've known some successful ones, the percentage of success in implants is poor. I consider implants risky. I do like the look of a good hairpiece on a man who needs or wants one because you have to look so closely to see them. Frankly, I think the cutting should be done at the wigmaker's. The top places will study you, make impressions, draw diagrams, and match the piece perfectly to the color of your hair, to the area to be covered, to those places where it should be thicker and thinner, shorter and longer. I'm balding a bit myself, and I don't mind. I think the bald look is becoming popular to some extent. But if a man feels he looks younger and better with the full head of hair he once had, I don't see why he shouldn't get a good piece styled to today's fashion. I don't see why men shouldn't do everything they can to make themselves look and feel better," Kenneth concludes.

Nor do I. Follow expert advice about your appearance. You will look and feel younger and better.

5

Dressing Right

Clothes are critical to anyone's appearance, of course. And a man can express his personality with the right choice of clothes. Accordingly, you can achieve a youthful appearance with the right choice of clothes.

It is helpful to have varied clothes for varied situations, but by choosing wisely you can make a small wardrobe work for many occasions. You should stick to the middle of the road and steer clear of extremes. A moderate style will last; fads come and go.

You don't have to have a high-fashion look to dress in fashion. You can go any way you want — to the highest fashion or the most casual fashion — and still stay in style. But if you're going to go in for fads, for things like turtlenecks and bell bottoms and leisure suits, your clothes are going to go out of style fast.

If you're going to look good, you're going to have to buy good clothes that are tailored to fit your figure. You may have to go to a good store because the tailors in most stores do not fit clothes to a man as well as they should be fit. Also, good fabrics will maintain their form better than poor fabrics. They will last longer and so, while you may spend more, you will get more for your money.

If you're going to look as good as possible, you'll have to be as slender as possible. If you're going to look youthful in a suit, you have to have a youthful figure. A youthful look is a trim, well-tailored, well-fit suit on a fit, trim body.

The style, cut, and color of clothes can conceal some excess weight. Or show weight excessively. A slender person can wear gaudy checks effectively, but they make a heavy man look heavier. Dark colors cover up weight a little. Stripes make a short person look taller. Short coats make a short person look taller. A little looser cut at the waist covers up some extra weight.

One key to looking good is neatness, of course. Because it is harder to fit a fatter fellow, his clothes seem to rumple and look messy faster than a thinner fellow's. But, whatever your figure, you can work at keeping your clothes clean and pressed and tidy.

Another key to looking good is posture. Clothes are designed to be worn in the erect position. They bag and crease if you do not stand erect. And most of us could improve our posture. We are not aware of how much we slouch and slump and how this drags the chest down, lets the stomach hang out, and pushes the rear end out.

Dinah Shore once attributed part of her youthful appearance to her good posture. You may not think about her posture when you look at her, but it's an important part of her look. If you think about it, few things are as important to our appearance as our posture.

I'm aware of my posture because I see myself on television. I tape my shows, then see myself on the screen later. I keep reminding myself to stand straight. Most performers have good posture because they have seen themselves on screen and have learned to stand straight.

Look closely at yourself in a three-way mirror like those they have in clothing stores. If you can afford it, buy yourself a three-way mirror. See yourself as others see you. I'll bet you'll begin to get your weight down and your posture up. Let your mirror be your screen.

Lift your head up, diminishing that double chin. Pull your shoulders back. Not too far back, but enough to bring your chest up and stomach in. Standing erect straightens your rear end, too. Stand, or sit, with your legs fairly close together, your feet straight.

You have to work at good posture. For a while you'll keep forgetting. After a while, it will come naturally.

You'll find you not only look better but feel better. The bones are aligned better. The muscles are being used better and will function better. You won't get as tired. Your clothes will fit better and look better.

Another key to the selection of clothes is the selection of color. The color of your clothes should coordinate with the color of your skin, eyes, and hair. People with dark hair, eyes, and skin should wear blues and grays. That's a general rule — and a safe one. Some of the muted shades in any of these colors can be worn by almost anyone. Next time you're buying a suit, try on a brown if you usually wear blue, and vice versa. Don't be afraid to experiment a little. People with light hair, eyes, and skin should wear browns and light greens.

I am not one of those people who think brown is wrong for nighttime wear. I think it's perfectly all right to wear brown shoes as long as you've got brown clothes on. I do flip when I see brown shoes with a blue suit. But, then, you shouldn't wear black shoes with a brown suit either.

I also cringe when I see white socks with anything but tennis shoes or running shoes. I think dark socks look best, socks that match the color of your shoes and pants. And I think the socks should be long and elasticized so that they stay up and cover your calves if your pants hike up. Baggy socks that fall down, and legs that are exposed when you sit down and cross your legs and your pants pull up, give you that good old country bumpkin look.

Your tie should blend with your coat. Golds with brown, grays with blues, and so forth. I don't like gaudy ties with too much design in them, but stripes are good. By the way, a gaudy tie won't make you look younger.

An eighteen-year-old often hikes his jacket sleeves up to his elbows, opens the collar of his shirt, and loosens the knot of his tie until he's wearing it at half-mast. An eighteen-year-old can get away with it. If you're thirty-eight, you can't. If you're wearing a tie, wear it all the way up, knotted neatly, and you'll look good.

In business, I often wear white shirts, and they're always in. White never really went out, even when colored shirts came in. And color is still in, though soft pastel colors rather than the gaudy colors we had for a while. More subtle designs are in than those we had for a while. I think a soft color in your shirt is youthful.

But don't try to fool the years. An older man is better off in lightweight, well-tailored slacks with a sports shirt open at the neck than in Bermuda shorts, just as an older woman is better off with well-fit slacks or a lightweight dress than in shorts or jeans.

The old guy in the black suit has given up. He'd look younger in a suit with a little color. Not a lot, a little.

The older man with his shirt open to his navel, wearing gold chains over a chest full of gray hair looks foolish, not younger. He'll look better with his shirt buttoned up.

I have a personal prejudice against jewelry on a man, but I guess there's nothing wrong with it. If you wear jewelry, I think you would be wise to wear fewer pieces and better pieces. It may make you look better, though not younger.

When I was younger and started to appear on television daily, I had a twenty-minute train commute from where I lived in suburban Drexel Hill to downtown Philadelphia. I didn't have much money, and I had only a few suits. But, every day, I stopped off at a one-day dry cleaners in downtown Drexel Hill to drop off one suit and pick up another I had dropped off the day before. That way

I kept changing, and everything I wore was clean and neat.

If I had only three suits to wear to business today, I would have (1) a dark blue suit, (2) a gray or brown suit, and (3) a light blue sports jacket with gray slacks or a light brown sports jacket with tan slacks. I would have four or five white shirts, two or three pastel-colored shirts, and two or three pastel sports shirts that could be worn with either the suits or the sports coat. Different-colored sports shirts and ties can make one suit or sports coat look different and keep your wardrobe flexible.

For some years now, I've gotten my clothes free for use on my show as part of the production costs of the show. This has built up my wardrobe. A performer is expected to wear different clothes from show to show, but he can't afford to buy a new suit for every appearance.

While I respect high-quality fabrics, I disagree with most stylists in that I believe in buying several less expensive suits or coats (as long as they are properly fitted) that are in style. That way, you can change off and always look fresh rather than own one better, more expensive suit that you have to wear all the time.

Obviously, if you buy less expensive clothes, you can buy more of them. You can buy clothes that are in fashion, and it will not be painful to put them away in a closet or even throw them away when they are out of fashion. Of course, you can't buy junk. You have to buy something in a good fabric that is well put together. You just don't have to buy the best.

I think if you wear one or two suits or sports outfits all the time, people will get sick of seeing you in them and you will tend to wear them until they're out of fashion. You have to have variety that suits the existing style.

However, most stylists will tell you that you are better off buying the best because it will wear better and look better longer and so give you more for your money in the long run. They say if you stick to moderate styles, you are better off with quality than quantity.

I would think it's up to the individual to decide what will work best for him in this situation. You should listen to the experts, then make up your own mind.

You may not have as many clothes as I do, but you can make the most of the clothes you do have. You may not need fashionable clothes in your work, but you can keep the clothes you do wear clean and neat. You should wear the clothes that fit your work. A fellow doesn't tend lawns in a suit and tie. But he may want to wear a suit and tie when he goes out at night.

Different parts of the country favor different styles. Businessmen in New

York do not dress as casually as those in California. You not only have to read the magazines that feature fashion; you have to look around you to get a grip on what's going in your area.

I'm a Californian now. I wear California kind of clothes — casual. I seldom wear suits to work. I usually wear a sports shirt and slacks, though I sometimes wear a sports coat. I seldom wear ties. In California you can wear a sports coat without a tie to most restaurants at night and be in fashion. I like casual clothes, but I choose stylish clothes that are not bright and gaudy.

But, on my shows and when I'm in New York, I usually wear a suit and tie. In business and in good restaurants in New York, men wear suits and ties. I have no objection to fitting the fashion wherever I am, and I think those who buck the trends tend to look foolish.

However, one thing that turns me off is the trend toward wearing labels instead of clothes. This used to be a failing of women, but now men have picked it up. Too many people worry more about buying a name brand than they do about buying the best they can find. All they're doing is becoming walking billboards for egocentric stylists who slap their names all over their products. A lot of teen-agers now are into this, too.

I wouldn't dare try to dress like a teen-ager, and I have no interest in the extremes of fashion. I try to keep up with fashions, not fads. Styles change, and you should change with them. That's youthful. Nothing betrays a person's age more than dressing the way he did when he was young. But you don't have to dress old.

You can get good clothes in keeping with your station in life. You're going to look foolish stepping out of your beat-up old car in a Gucci belt and Gucci shoes. Everyone will know that's all you have and you're just trying to put on a show.

To get a cross-section of expert advice I have turned to Bruce Geller, executive vice-president of Botany 500 Clothes in New York, and Marge Swenson of the Fashion Academy of Costa Mesa, California, which does not sell clothes but consults with clients on the right clothes for them to wear.

My experts differ on some specifics but tend to agree on basics. In any event, they give good advice, which should guide you in making your decisions on dress.

Bruce says, "In buying clothes, you should consider the intrinsic value of your investment, especially in these difficult times. I believe you are better off buying quality instead of quantity because you will get more for your money and it will cost you less in the long run. You can dress up a basic suit and make it look different with the right choice of appropriate accessories. I consider accessories as important as the suit or sports outfit."

Marge, who is one of many women who have a trained eye for what looks good on a man, says, "We use a word most men will understand — amortization. It applies to clothes, too. The most expensive clothes eventually should repay your investment. The least expensive may not, though you have spent less. What you want to consider is the cost per wearing, as well as the pleasure you get from the outfit. The better suits will last longer, look better for longer, and give you more wearings than lesser suits.

"They say only the very rich and the very poor wear out their clothes. The very rich buy such high-quality clothes they last a long time and they tend to wear them until they fall apart. The very poor buy such low-quality clothes they tend to fall apart in a short time. But most people can afford to buy clothes that will last awhile and look good awhile and replace them as they show wear.

"Although price is not the only criterion to consider in purchasing a suit or coat — good suits today start at about $350, coats at about $200 — I believe you are wise to go for quality. A good natural fiber, such as wool, will mold itself to your body; synthetics will not, though synthetics mixed with wool will give your clothes a little longer life. Natural fibers look better and feel better.

"A worsted wool suit or coat will last five to fifteen years, a synthetic perhaps only three years. One item you can save on is slacks. Because they get heavy wear, you might be wise to wear synthetic fiber slacks at about $25 or $30 a pair and replace them as they wear out, but you would still not be unwise to go up to as much as $150 for a fine, natural fiber pair."

Bruce says that if he could afford only two or three suits, they would be wool or a polyester blend: "The most popular, dollar for dollar, is a blend of 55 percent Dacron polyester and 45 percent worsted wool. This is considered the 'classic' blend. If I could have only one suit it would be a ten- to ten-and-a-half-ounce polyester or worsted suit that could be worn year round. If a fellow can also afford a spring wardrobe, nothing is more comfortable than an eight- to eight-and-a-half-ounce polyester and wool tropical suit. This might be a year-round suit for someone in southern California or a tropical climate.

"If I could have only three suits, they would be a navy blue pinstripe, a solid gray, and a solid brown in moderate styles. The darkest suit is best for a young man going on a job interview. I believe a young man should wear his best suit, a dress shirt, and a subdued tie to an interview, for any job, no matter what he will be doing or wearing on that job.

"If I couldn't have a more extensive wardrobe, I would substitute a navy blue blazer for the gray or brown suit, with gray solid slacks to go with it. Every man should have this set. Whether he is young or old. It has a youthful look and fits many occasions. Black is old-looking and out. Brown is wrong for nighttime wear. Brown shoes are acceptable only with brown suits."

Marge disagrees with Bruce here. She says, "There is nothing wrong whatsoever with brown for evening wear. This idea started in New York and possibly with a very suspect survey of New Yorkers, who tend to have a lot of dark-colored men in the population.

"A man should dress according to his skin and eyes and hair coloring, working a lot with 'neutrals.' While we get more specific in individual consultations with each particular client, there are two broad categories. One is those with dark coloring who look best in dark blue to gray, who can accessorize them with shirts and ties in all shades of blue, spruce green, and rich maroon, and with black shoes. The other is those of lighter color, such as brown-haired and blond people, who look best in a basic color group that ranges from dark brown to camel and beige and who should wear

brown, gold, rust, or greens in their ties
and belts, and brown shoes.

"A man should dress to his coloring,
and those suited to browns should not
bow down to a New York prejudice
against browns. But I do have a prejudice
against black clothes. They're forbidding.
They're for funerals and ministers.

"Every man needs at least one suit,
and it should be of a medium color that
suits his color group. It should be
neither dark nor light but in the middle
of his group. It will work for job inter-
views, weddings, all special occasions, as
well as business. The fabric should be of
a hard, flat finish of worsted wool or a
polyester-wool blend that will wear well,
and of a muted, textured pattern such as
a thin stripe, a hounds-tooth or a her-
ringbone that will not show wrinkles. If
he can afford one or two other suits, they
can be of more extreme dark or light
colors in his color group. The second
should be darker and plain, the third
lighter with a pattern. Gabardine, flan-
nels, and twills work well.

"Frankly, if a man wears suits to work,
he should have at least five of them so
that he looks different every day and his
suits have a chance to relax and recover
from each wearing. No suit should be
worn two days in a row. On the other
hand, no man needs more than ten suits.
If he has more, he has made poor
choices or had poor fittings. He won't be

wearing all those suits, and they'll be wasting away in his closet. Many men cannot afford five suits, of course, and they can get by with two or three if they choose them wisely.

"A sports coat of a medium color in a man's group would be a wise substitute for a third suit. If possible, a man should have two or three sports coats of various colors within his group. My first choice for the darker man would be a navy blue coat, for the lighter man a camel coat. Two slacks in colors that blend with the coat will enable each coat to do double duty.

"It looks best if a man puts the plainest and darkest patterns on the largest part of his body. If he is a well-built or big man with broad shoulders and a large chest, he should wear dark, plain-colored coats with bright or patterned slacks. Smaller, thinner men are better off with brighter or patterned coats and darker, plainer slacks."

The expert from Fashion Academy adds, "I like vests on men. Suits with vests make those suits both businesslike and dressy when you wear the vest. Vests have impact. I also like sweaters on men. Most men could afford two — a vest-sweater type, which can be worn with sports shirt and slacks, and which, when worn with a suit, changes the whole look of the suit; and a cardigan that can be worn in place of a sports coat.

"The man should have three or four long-sleeved and short-sleeved sports shirts, but all business shirts should be long-sleeved. Short-sleeved business shirts carry the connotation of the blue-collar worker. An executive wearing a long-sleeved shirt can roll up his sleeves at work and still look like an executive.

"The appropriate leisure look is not as trendy as the business look. Jeans are in and always will be in. But they should fit snugly and many men with big bellies or big behinds cannot wear snug jeans and look good. Some of the major jeans manufacturers turn out jeans that are styled poorly and fit only the very slim well. You do not get jeans or shorts tailored to your form the way you do suits and slacks, so you have to try them on and select them carefully. Bermuda shorts are back; but short, heavy men cannot wear them well. The average man would be better off in lightweight tailored slacks and sports shirts.

"There are two types of sports shirts that call for special consideration. Those that have a banded collar will stand up in a perky look and can be worn well open, standing up inside the jacket. Those that do not have a banded collar lay down and can be worn well open, laying outside the jacket. In dress shirts, white or off-white shirts are always in style. A man should have a couple of plain white shirts and a couple of white-on-white shirts. Only a really dark person can wear chalk white well.

"Men should have some dress shirts in colors, but pale colors are safest. Ice tones are in — pale blue shirts with dark blue coats, canary yellow shirts with dark brown coats. A man should never wear dark shirts or these white-collar, dark-body shirts to business. The eye goes to the lightest color, so you want a light-colored shirt. A little pattern is all right, although less for business than for evening wear.

"There is no such thing as a wash-and-wear shirt, by the way. If a dress shirt is going to look good, you might spray a little starch on the collar, cuffs, and upper front, at least, and use an iron on these areas to give the shirt a fresh, crisp look.

"Ties should be selected to blend with the color of your coat and shirt. Men in the darker group can go to blues, grays, blue-reds or true reds, perhaps some yellows. The light group can go to golds, yellows, greens, tomato reds. Unless you have a lot of ties, safe patterns are preferred. Small patterns or narrow stripes. Bright colors and broad patterns tend to destroy the sense of style you should have established with your clothing.

"Belts and shoes should be the same color. Belts should be leather, thin, probably plain. Shoes should be leather. The smoother the leather, the dressier the shoe, while patterned shoes with thicker soles are best for business. Interestingly, patent leather is businesslike on a man, sporty on a woman. As for jewelry, I think you can overdo it. Most men look best in simple, handcrafted, light pieces."

The man from Botany 500 says, "Accessories are the things that make a suit effective or ineffective. I am not talking about jewelry. I think a lot of jewelry looks out of place on a man. If an older man thinks a lot of jewelry makes him look younger, he is fooling himself. But ties, shirts, belts, socks, and shoes should be carefully chosen to compliment your basic attire and make it look its best.

"In shirts, stripes are in, prints are out. Whites are always in, but a little color remains in, too. Long-sleeved, lightweight shirts are very good. Shorter collars are coming in, and button-down collars — the preppy look — are coming back. Button-down collars go well with coats with natural, soft shoulders. These shoulders are in. Narrower ties are in, but not string ties. About two or three inches in width. One must remember that as collars get narrower, ties have to be narrower. The color and pattern of the tie should be subdued and match the coat and shirt. The wrong shirt and tie can make a $600 suit look like a $100 suit.

"Woolen and argyle socks in grays

and blues are very popular. Cotton and nylon socks go well in the spring. The argyle socks today come in subtle mixtures of colors that can be blended well with the color of your pants. In shoes, the casual look is in. Slip-ons and loafers, some with tassels, are in. Even cowboy boots are becoming fashionable for all situations. The hard shiny look is out. Suede is acceptable, especially in the fall. I think the Italian, narrow look took its toll on men's feet, and I'm happy to see it going out of style.

"Men should not go in for gimmickry. Leisure suits, for example, lasted about a year and dated many a wardrobe. A man can compromise effectively by not going for extremes. I think the men's clothing industry is stabilizing anyway. Changes in fashion are coming slow and are slight. Some years ago, five-inch lapels were in. Now, three-inch lapels are in. I doubt we'll go back to two-inch lapels. A man is safest buying a lapel three to three and a half inches wide, and he will stay in fashion for a long time. Every fine manufacturer provides clothes in these compromise styles, and a man can find them in every fine store.

"Every man is different, and when he tries on a suit in a store, it should say something to him about himself. He should be able to say, 'This is me.' He should insist that a tailor take care with the fitting of his suits, coats, and pants.

Heavy men shouldn't wear plaids. Short men should wear stripes. The pattern and fit of a suit should be selected to play up a man's strong points and play down his weak points.

"A man should insist on buying a suit that a tailor will take care to fit him properly. The clothes that suit a man's coloring and personality and that fit him properly are the ones that make him look best and most youthful." Bruce Geller concludes.

Marge Swenson says, "We also classify people by their personality types. There are, just to name a few, businessmen, romantics, outdoor sorts. There are definite differences. The natural, outdoor sort of man can make a suggestive comment or joke to a woman and she'll laugh because she feels he's joking. The romantic type makes the same sort of crack, and a woman will be offended because she believes he is serious.

"The type of person a man is affects the sort of clothes he wears. The romantic man can wear exotic clothes and get away with them better than others can. The outdoorsman can wear casual clothes and get away with them better than others can. The businessman cannot get away with jewelry the way a romantic can, while an outdoors sort just can't be bothered. Flamboyants can wear fads.

"Your coloring, your personality type,

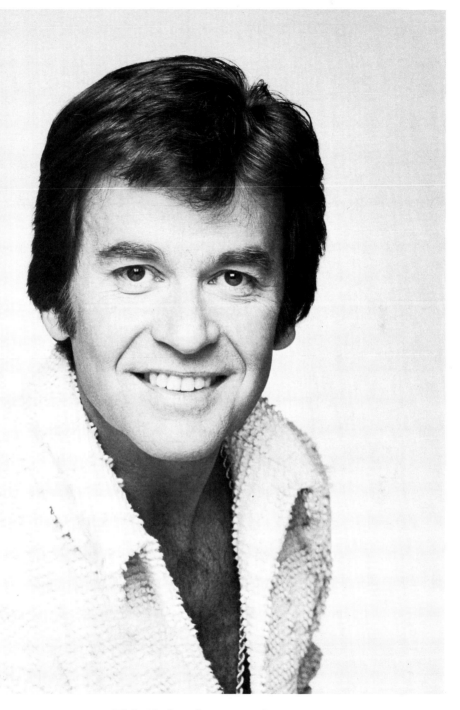

**Dick Clark today at age 50.
Eat your heart out, Robert Redford.**

I didn't get just a wife; I got
two dogs of somewhat
different type, color, shape,
and size. Here, one greets me
affectionately, but I don't kiss
back.

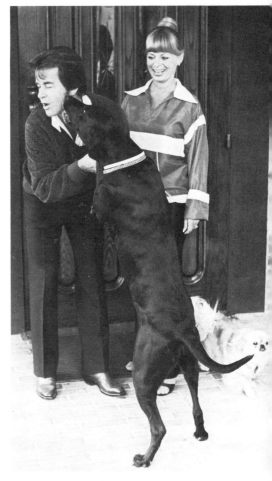

Here I am in the spring of
1980 with my wife, Kari.

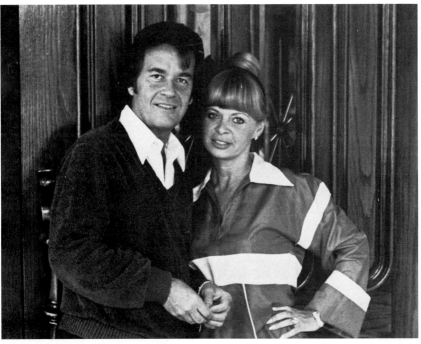

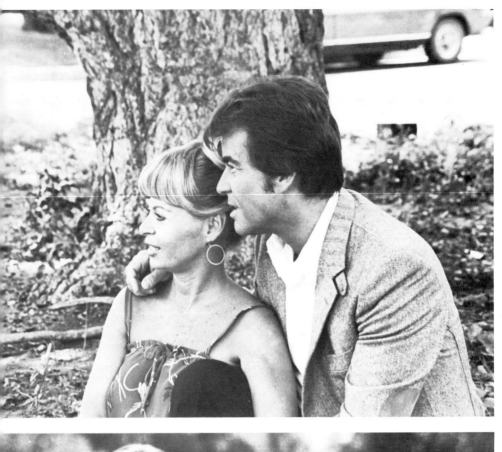
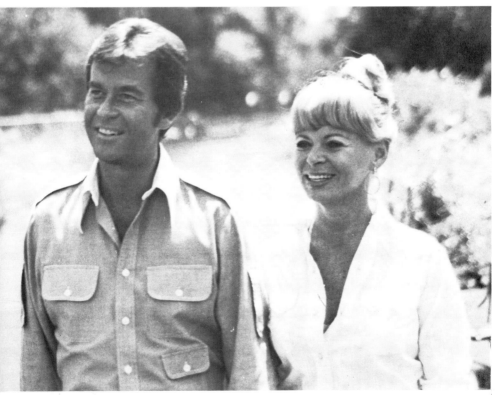

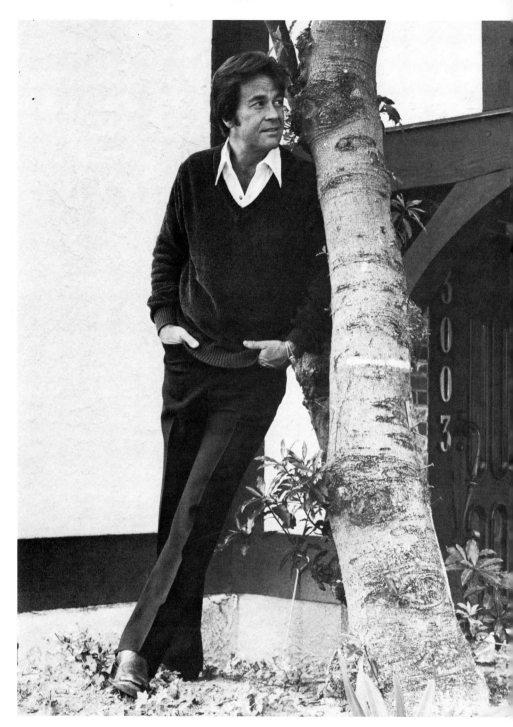

Stealing a breath of fresh air outside my offices.

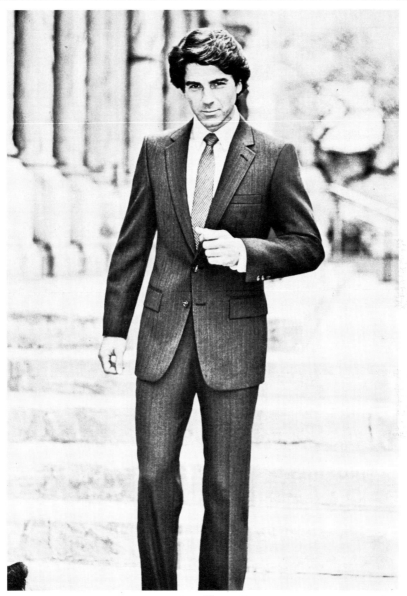

The Bentley from Botany '500'®—tailored for the man who likes to look up-to-date without being faddish. The slightly shaped jacket with squared shoulders gives this classic suit a sophisticated appearance that's proper in almost any situation. *Photo:* Bob Barclay, N.Y. *Model:* Patrick Zack, represented by Ford Men, N.Y.

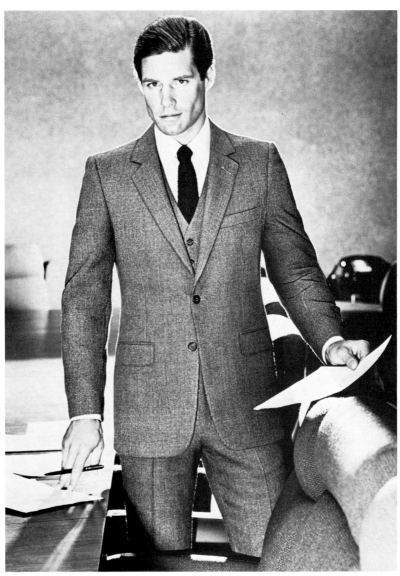

The Cartier® Executive from Botany '500'®—a European-shaped suit that's tailored for the American body so the mature man can look trim and feel comfortable at the same time. Its shaped-shoulder styling and pinstripe fabrication make it the ideal suit for both professional and special occasions. *Photo:* Bob Barclay, N.Y. *Model:* Scott Webster, represented by Ford Men, N.Y.

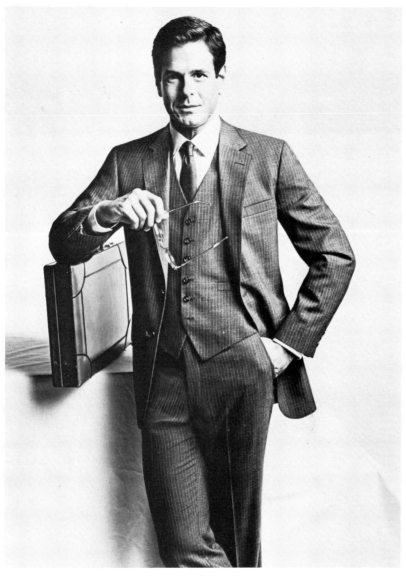

The Chase from Botany '500'® is the ultimate in traditional business suits. The relaxed natural shoulders and understated details give it a timeless look that will keep it up-to-date for years to come. *Photo:* Bob Barclay, N.Y. *Model:* Richard Smith, represented by Ford Men, N.Y.

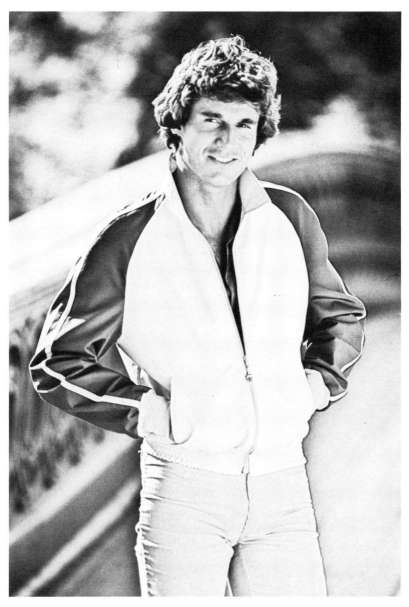

McGregor® designed this fully lined lightweight jacket for the active man who thinks sportswear should work on the field or off. *Photo:* Michelle Barclay, N.Y. *Model:* Patrick St.Clair, represented by Ford Men, N.Y.

where you live and what you do, your life style — all affect your choice of clothes. But all can keep in fashion by keeping in the middle of the road. If real wide lapels are in, get yours a little narrower. If real narrow lapels are in, get yours a little wider. You can always get the width you want in good stores. Shorter, narrower, but not narrow lapels are in right now. Shorter, narrower, but not narrow shirt collars are in now. Straight, stovepipe pants are in. Narrower, but not narrow ties are in. Three-inch collars and three-inch ties are in. A tip many men can use: The narrower and shorter the coat lapel or collar, the narrower the tie must be and the smaller the knot. The big Windsor tie won't go with today's style. You have to tie a half-Windsor or some sort of tight knot.

"While the cycle in women's clothes runs about three years for major changes, that for men's clothes runs longer, about five to seven years, and I think it's stabilizing now. It takes a flamboyant type to wear faddish clothes. Only the very young can get away with the sort of things they sell in the mod boutiques. Those clothes are expensive, and I don't know how many young men can afford them. They go out of style very fast. Many of the extreme things they sell for a short time never really are in style. The older man is kidding himself if he thinks he's going to look younger in

these extremes. He can't get away with
them.

"The youngest look is slender, lithe,
form-fitting. The average mature man
cannot get away with this. Let's face it,
the most youthful look is the slender
look. But a man can be as youthful as
possible by being as slender as possible
and by having his clothes cut to make
him look as slender as possible. A man
will look slimmer and more youthful if
his coats are shaped well on the sides,
under his arms, through to the waist. A
double-vented suit often will look slimmer. But a double-breasted suit, while in,
is out for the heavier man. Double-
breasted suits do look best on most
men."

The expert from the Fashion Academy points out, "The thing we have found
is that most suits, no matter how fine,
have not been fine-fit to the individual.
We have unskilled clothiers selling suits
and coats and pants and very few well-
trained and skilled custom tailors. You
have to seek out skilled clothiers and
tailors. Suits should fit snug. Sports
coats, too, though they can be a little
looser.

"Most men buy suits too large, as if
they want to play ball in them. But, usually, they take their coats off even to drive
a car. They will be seen in their suits
standing in an office, at a party, at a
dance, and the suit should fit snugly to

their form. When a woman touches the sleeve, she should feel flesh. She should not have to press through the fabric to find a man's arm.

"The rule of thumb that a coat should extend to the knuckles doesn't take into account the length of the man's arm. The coat should carry to the crotch. However, a slightly shorter coat will make a shorter man look taller, a slightly longer coat will make a taller man look shorter.

"You have got to seek out quality tailoring if you are going to look your best in any clothes. Buy and wear good clothes that are not flagrantly out of fashion and that fit your shape, personality, and coloring and take care of your clothes and you will look younger and better," Marge concludes.

I agree. And I do not know many men who would not look better by dressing better. Slimming down would help most men dress better, but choosing good clothes in keeping with current fashion and getting those that fit you and are fit to you will do a lot for you. You can take years off your age by dressing right.

6

Exercise
and Diet

I love to eat and I hate to diet. I love all
kinds of food — good for you, bad for
you, and otherwise. I even love to
cook. I'm married to a lady who loves to
eat and is no help to me whatsoever
where food is concerned.

I'm not fat, but I could be in a fast
minute. I fight it every hour of every day.
Kari is round in all the right places. She's
not fat, but she could be. Most of the
fights we have are over food. We fight for
the last piece on the plate.

One of these years, maybe when I'm
off the air, we'll let loose. We'll turn into

those two people in *Alice in Wonder-
land* — Tweedle Dee and Tweedle
Dum — and roll around the house.

We've made a pact. When one of us
dies of terminal obesity, the other will
cover it up, claiming death came from a
heart attack, an attack by killer bees, or a
fall from favor . . . or somewhere!

Diet and exercise go hand in hand,
like drinking and falling down. The only
thing I like less than dieting is exercising.
It's easier to stop eating than it is to start
running. I like to work, but I don't like to
work up a sweat. Games bore me.

As a boy, I thought I was athletic. I
went out for a lot of teams. Swimming
and football were two. I didn't make any.
I did set a school record for push-ups
and came close in sit-ups, at good old
A. B. Davis High in Mount Vernon. I still
sit, but I don't do sit-ups. I do swim. I
ran until my arches fell.

I'm 5 feet 9 inches tall and weigh 158
pounds. That's not too bad. I don't look
too bad on television. But all it takes is
three or four pounds, and I look bad. I
step on the scales whenever I have the
strength. As soon as I see the needle
inching around 160, I step off.

Fat isn't beautiful. Neither is skinny.
There's a happy medium.

I'll eat anything as long as it's the
wrong thing. I like all kinds of food as
long as it's junk food. I love Italian food.
That's not junk food, but I'm an Italian

food junkie. I can put the pasta away like you've seldom seen.

I love meat and hate fish. Naturally. The one that's better for me I like less. I do like chicken, which isn't too bad. I like fruits and vegetables, which is good. I like undercooked or raw vegetables, which is great.

I love chocolate, which is terrible for you. I'm a chocolataholic just like I'm a workaholic. I'm convinced there's a connection between the two. Chocolate provides quick energy. With energy, you work well. Chocolate is a narcotic. You can get hooked on it, like any drug. Periodically, I cut it out. I go cold turkey. There are times I hide chocolate around the house the way an alcoholic conceals bottles of booze, so there'll always be some when I want it.

OK, if you know you're weak, you have to do something about it. You like to eat, but the more you eat, the less you like yourself. The fatter you are, the worse you look. I hate it when my clothes get tight on me. It makes me want to do something about it.

I make it a rule that the minute I hit 160 pounds, I stop eating. I cut it out. All of it. That's my secret. I go cold turkey. It's 160 for me. It's probably another figure for you. But you have to draw the line somewhere for yourself, and stick to it. You can't just look at yourself, frown, and say, "Tomorrow." It has to be today.

Vanity is only one reason for keeping the extra pounds off. Survival is another. Statistically, it's clear that the more overweight you are, the greater your risk of dying from heart trouble, strokes, and such. Sugar-rich foods feed diabetes. Fatty foods increase the cholesterol, and that clogs the arteries. The cholesterol problem is being rethought by some scientists, but I think you should play it cool where cholesterol is concerned.

Clearly, drugs are destructive. I see a lot of it around. From cocaine to pill-popping. It seems to be the "in" thing in Hollywood and on Broadway. Too many people with too much money and too much fame are looking for something different to do for kicks.

Narcotics and pills have done in a lot of stars, from Marilyn Monroe to Janis Joplin. Most performers are smart enough to steer clear of the stuff. I'm one of them. It's stupid to get on drugs of any sort. I don't have to tell you. You know it.

I did smoke tobacco for years, but I gave it up about ten years ago. A relative died of lung cancer at a time I had developed a bad cough. It scared some sense into me. I went cold turkey. You probably can, too, if you want it enough. If you feel you can't, try one of the commercial programs. Some use methods that may be distasteful, but any method that works is worthwhile. It's clear by now that cigarettes can't do you any good.

I used to drink a lot of alcohol. Too much. Partly that was because of personal troubles. My first marriage broke up in the worst way. A man's wife called me up to tell me her husband was running around with my wife. The fellow was supposed to be my friend. He wasn't.

After the divorce I was depressed and turned to drink. Straight vodka, mainly. I came to my shows with hangovers, did them with headaches. I came close to becoming an alcoholic. And an ex-star. This was in late 1961, early 1962.

Friends straightened me out. They talked to me straight. Especially Connie Francis and Bobby Darin. They made me see I had friends. And a lot to live for. I stopped heavy drinking. Lately, I've turned to drinking wine socially, rather than the hard stuff, and I keep it light. But one man's light drinking is another man's heavy drinking. You have to know yourself.

Hard drinking is as big a problem with young people as hard drugs. But I don't think it's the young thing to do. It's the dumb thing to do. It's easier to kick your youth than it is to kick drugs and drink. They both make you old fast.

Cutting down on drink also saved me a lot of calories. When you come right down to it, saving on calories is the only way to save your figure. I've tried every diet that's come along. Some seem to work for a while. Some may work, period. Some are ridiculous. In the final analysis, any good diet is simply a system for cutting down on your caloric intake, so you can do what any diet can do by cutting down on the calories.

When I hit 160 pounds, I throw away my fork. I go on a two-day or three-day fast. You should check with your doctor before going on a fast, but I do it and it works for me. It's hard at first, but, for me, cutting out food entirely is easier than cutting down on food.

I take vitamins every day. I drink a lot of water. If I get too hungry for comfort, I drink a little juice, preferably vegetable juice. Otherwise, on my fasts, I am cold turkey.

No, I don't eat cold turkey.

I know some doctors will disagree, but I find that the vitamins seem to keep my strength up. I don't feel weak, in any event. The fast seems to shrink my stomach so that soon my desire for food goes down. And it shows on the scales. It helps me lose a little weight fast, which encourages me to continue. We all need encouragement.

What we need more than anything else is the desire to be trim. It's strictly up to you how much you want to be in shape. I want it. That's me up there on the screen. And in the mirror.

When my fast is finished, it's easier for me to get on a good, balanced diet than it otherwise would have been because I'm happy to be eating anything again.

Any doctor will tell you that a good balanced diet is the best thing you can do for your body. My idea of a balanced diet is "passion and pleasure," which is what I call a dish called Pasta Primavera. That's noodles mixed with vegetables and seasoned with garlic. I love garlic. I consider garlic not only sensational seasoning but a cure-all for what ails you. Medical science is just turning on to this. Some doctors will tell you that garlic is great medicine, a fine health food, a sort of "super vegetable" with a lot of vitamin value.

Dr. William Klein laughs and says, "I don't know about garlic, but I'll admit there's talk about its being beneficial for some things. I don't even know about all vitamins, but do prescribe some of them in certain instances. If someone is found to have pernicious anemia, I prescribe Vitamin B_{12}. But if someone says he lacks pep and energy, I won't fill him full of B_{12} shots. If someone is found to be low in iron, I prescribe iron. But if I can't prove that deprivation of a specific vitamin leads to a specific deficiency, I won't prescribe the vitamin.

"My kids take multivitamins with fluoride more for the fluoride than for the vitamins. I believe there is sufficient evidence that fluoride is good for your teeth. But there is insufficient evidence that most artificial vitamins do anything for anything. I can get all the vitamins I want free, and I don't use them.

"The body throws off half the vitamins you take anyway. For the most part, taking excessive vitamins won't hurt you. However, vitamins A and D have been found to be harmful in some cases. Too much vitamin D, for example, seems to result in the development of kidney stones and starts a string of other problems. Except for teeth and bone development in young people, I don't believe healthy people need artificial vitamins if they have a healthy diet. With the help of a good, balanced diet, their bodies produce all the vitamins they need. Of course, we all know the average diet of the average person consists largely of garbage."

Bill says, "I'm a meat and potatoes doctor, but where diet is concerned I believe in a lot of fish and fowl. There is some controversy over cholesterol. This may be because cholesterol consists of several things. We consider that there is good cholesterol and bad cholesterol. Elevated levels of triglyceride count in your cholesterol indicates you need to reduce your fatty intake. Cholesterol can coat the linings of your arteries and narrow them down dangerously. But the fact is, the body produces two-thirds of our cholesterol. So, in cutting down, we are dealing with only about one-third. Clearly we would be wise to cut down on fatty foods, but unless a patient is found to have a problem, I don't tell him to cut down on meat and dairy foods.

"Obviously, a balanced diet consists of food from the four food groups — meats, fruits and vegetables, dairy products, and breads and cereals. It is a matter of how much from each. The body needs both carbohydrates and protein. Carbohydrates are complex sugars and starches the body converts into fuel. How much you need depends on how active you are and how much energy you need. The excess turns into fat. Proteins do not provide energy, but they build and repair muscle tissue, regulate the body's functions, and provide vitamins, antibodies, and enzymes necessary to health. Proteins are provided in meat and fish, milk, eggs, rice, corn, potatoes, peanuts. Vegetarians prove you can do without meat. You can do without eggs. But experts have found that you can't do without all these things. High-protein diets are not bad, but they're rarely balanced, and that's bad. The body also needs minerals and vitamins."

Concludes Dr. Klein, "All a person needs for a balanced diet is common sense. Unfortunately, few of us seem to have it, or, at least, to exercise it. The common misconception I find in my work is that people think there is a doctor, treatment, or pill to do for them what they are too weak to do for themselves. The overweight person prefers a pill to the painful, long-term task of reducing what he eats and the unappetizing prospect of changing what he eats. I'm not a great fan of fad diets. Those that work do so because the dieter is taking in less calories, one way or another. Most fad diets do not work because they are unappetizing. A lot of people go on diets. Few stay on them. We know weight can pose critical problems to our health. I don't know if it will make a person look younger, but if he or she wants to live longer, a good diet is desirable."

Well, Doctor Bill, that's laying it on the line. Ask for advice, and it lands on you. Let me lay this on you: Between marriages, I was trying to make love to a nice lady and I couldn't get an erection. It was embarrassing and frightening. Here I was forty or so, and I felt like I was fading fast. There was distracting noise next door, but I laid the blame on age when I couldn't accommodate the nice lady. I took a real head trip. I'd heard about vitamin E working wonders sexually, so I stocked up. I haven't failed since, so I guess it hasn't failed me. Frankly, I think it is in my head, not in the vitamin. But I think if taking a vitamin makes you feel better or more confident, even if it is all in your head, it's worth it, as long as you don't overdo it. I have such good feelings about vitamin E, I've even broken capsules and rubbed the stuff on facial blemishes — with good results.

I take vitamin B-complex, and I do have a lot of pep and energy. I used to take a mixture of vitamins I made up myself. I finally succeeded in getting a company to put together a combination that's medically sound and one that seems to work for me. It has the Dick Clark endorsement. I take this special combination every day. It contains multiple vitamins and minerals and Vitamin E. E is often referred to as the anti-aging vitamin. It fights the bad effects of smog and pollution. Laboratory tests indicate that Vitamin E – treated cells live longer. Draw your own conclusion.

I take extra vitamin C, though I still get colds, but fewer of them, and, it seems to me, less harsh ones. I for one believe in vitamins every day, but not to excess. I've taken vitamins every day for over forty years. Maybe they don't help, but if they're not bad for you, why not? I endorse vitamins and believe they have helped me personally. I think if you don't eat properly, or are dieting, the vitamins you take will be working for you.

I do listen to my doctors, and I do try to do what they tell me to do. I am told that exercise is a hard way to lose even a little weight, but that exercise combined with diet will help you lose weight. And by itself exercise is beneficial to your body in many ways. It promotes good circulation throughout your body, builds up the capacity of your heart and lungs, and tones up your muscles.

I am told that a calorie is a unit of heat, a measurement of the energy in different foods. In our daily activities we burn up this energy. We usually take in more calories than we can burn up, and what is left turns to fat. The average person is 10 to 20 percent overweight. If you are 10 percent overweight, you are twice as apt to develop high blood pressure, three times as apt to develop diabetes, and four times as apt to have heart trouble as if you are at a normal weight. If you are twice again as overweight, you are more than twice again as apt to have these problems. At 20 percent overweight, you are regarded as obese.

I am around my normal body weight for my height and age, so I suppose I look younger than some other people because most others are not. I am told that every pound of excess weight you have represents about 4,000 calories that you must burn off if you are going to lose that pound. A full hour's hard run burns up less than 1,000 calories. An hour of tennis less than 500 calories. An hour's brisk walk only a little more than 200.

The average person needs 2,000 to 3,000 calories a day to function well, but takes in closer to 4,000. So he gains weight. He has to cut to around 2,000 to 2,500 calories a day to lose weight.

You can't eat too much cake or candy if you're going to stay under 2,500 calories a day. A small piece of cake can represent 100 to 300 calories. You simply have to cut down or cut out starches and sweets. A glass of a soft drink or beer is 100 calories. A glass of whiskey or wine may be 150. A little portion of lobster may be 200. An ordinary portion of french fries is 200. An ordinary portion of spaghetti is more than 200.

But a cup of bouillon is only 5 calories. A piece of celery is only 5. A portion of carrots is only about 25. A small portion of fish is only about 30 calories, and a small portion of chicken only about 50. A cup of coffee or tea without sugar or cream is only about 2 calories, but if you add a sliver of pie, you're adding 200 calories.

Clearly, you have to rethink your eating habits if you're going to revitalize your body and get to looking good. You are not going to be able to exercise away that spaghetti and pie, that hamburger and fries, unless that's all you eat all day. And if that's all you eat all day, your body is going to age away and break down. If you want to fit into those sleek slacks, you'd better bear down. Do it, don't talk about it. Too many people do too little and talk too much. Cut down on your eating and step up your exercise.

Clearly, exercise helps you stay young. So how do you explain me? Chemistry! I do swim as often as I can. I really like swimming. And I'm told it's one of the best exercises for the average person, even though it does not take a lot of energy and does not burn up a lot of calories. It does use every muscle in your body and does build up your heart and lungs.

For the last three years, I have had one of those exercycle contraptions. I hate it. Every day I look at it and wish somehow, mysteriously, it would disappear. In any case, I force myself to ride it, usually in the morning, until I huff and puff appropriately. I usually watch television while this is going on because, quite frankly, I find exercise boring. I know it's good for you, but I full out hate it.

I used to run, but running on soft sand at the beach can be dangerous, and I did some damage to my feet. Running is considered good exercise, but running on hard city sidewalks can be bad for the arches and shins. Many people are doing damage to their legs these days. Jogging is a craze, but experts tell me that it jars the whole skeletal structure and that outright running really is better for you. Not sprinting, but running a mile or

more at ten minutes a mile or less, building up your distance and speed as you
go.

The actor Bruce Dern, who was a
competitive runner a part of his life and
has been a dedicated runner almost all
his life, a fellow who does not miss a day
of his life without doing some real running, says, "I don't believe there is such a
thing as jogging. It's just slow running.
When I see my forty-five-year-old agent
running, I figure he thinks he's jogging,
but I know he's just running slowly and
will run faster if he keeps on running.
Short sprints hurt much more than slow
long-distance runs. You can build yourself up to where you can run slowly a
long way without its hurting too much.
But I run fast and hard, and it hurts. I
hear a lot about the euphoria of running,
but I've never felt it. I just feel pain. I run
because I believe it's good for you. And
the only reason I don't take time off from
it is because it hurts like hell when I try
to get back to it."

Frank O'Neill, a long-time major
league athletic trainer around L.A., says,
"Running is by far the best exercise. It
burns up the most calories and builds
up your body best. The longer you run,
the better it is for you. Bicycling is next
best. If you do it hard, it will do you a lot
of good. Swimming is very good for you.
Handball and racquetball are better than
tennis and skiing because you have to

work harder at them. In tennis, singles is better than doubles, again because you have to work harder. Golf and bowling don't do you a lot of good because you don't run and you don't work hard. If you ride a golf cart on the course, forget it."

Frank is in favor of *any* exercise rather than no exercise. He says, "I believe any activity you pursue that requires you to move around and use your muscles is good for you, and I think everyone of every age should do something. Walking is not as good as running, but it sure beats doing nothing. Skipping rope is super. Child's play? Try it sometime. It's difficult, but if you can recapture your childhood skills, it's fun and beneficial. It loosens up the body and gets the juices boiling. And it's terrific for rhythm and timing. Girls used to skip rope more than boys, of course. But men can do it as well as women. Boxers do it.

"Isometrics are very good, but more for the muscle tone than for all-around health. They're simple to do and especially easy in the office. Every few seconds you can grab are good. You can even do isometrics while talking on the telephone. Press the palms of your two hands together hard, using the resistance of your muscles to make your muscles work. Lock your fingers and try to pull your hands apart. Sit at a desk and push down on the desk, or try to lift your chair up while you're sitting in it. Build up a little bit at a time. These are explosive exercises, and they can strain the heart.

"Simple calisthenics not only are good for your physical condition but are a good warm-up for your day, your work, and your play. And you should warm up before exercise to loosen up your muscles and skeletal structure and avoid injuries. Not just sit-ups and push-ups, but stretching routines. Shake your arms and legs. Stretch from tiptoes and try to reach your fingertips to the ceiling, and bend with straight knees to try to touch your toes. With hands on hips, rotate your upper body and head as far around as you can. Sit down and stretch to touch your toes, slowly, holding it.

"Take ten minutes or more every morning to stretch and loosen your muscles and get your circulation going. Your body will benefit, and you'll feel better and be able to work better. And try to get in some exercise at least every day because it's too dangerous to lay off all week and subject your body to excessive strain on the weekend. If you haven't been active, start slowly and build up gradually. If you are active, stick to it. Professional athletes last longer these days because they've found that age doesn't slow them as much as they thought, and if they stay at their sport and keep a positive attitude about it, they can go on and on. A Gordie Howe was still playing big-league hockey in his fifties because he stayed in shape and just kept going. You can be younger than your years if you get in shape and keep going," concludes Frank O'Neill.

Gotcha, Frank. I'm going out for a hockey team today. But to avoid danger I won't do anything physical this weekend because I haven't done anything physical all week. Other than having sex. And I consider sex a physical activity that is beneficial to both body and mind. I'm sure I'm far from the best in bed, but I have found I'm better in bed when I'm better off physically, when I'm fit and healthy. And I feel I have a youthful attitude about the physical activity of sex. I believe sincerely in "more is better" in this department. More on sex later.

One nice sort of sexual activity is dancing — boy-girl, man-woman dancing. I'd be nuts if I didn't recommend dancing as an exercise, and Frank agrees with me that any active dance is strenuous exercise. Some of the dances we've had on our show sure have to be considered strenuous.

We use slow and fast dances on "Bandstand." Early on, fast dances took over. We started with the jitterbug and Lindy Hop, but soon were into the Bop, the Stroll, the Shake, the Walk, the Shag, the Twist, the Pony, the Watusi, the Fly, the Jerk, the Fish, and so forth.

If you don't think they're strenuous exercise, try them. Any of them. The Twist used to shake you to pieces. I was scared to death of it when I first saw a couple of kids doing it on our show. The old folks complain that the man and woman aren't in each other's arms in dances like this, but if the kids had as much as touched while twisting their pelvises, we'd have been arrested.

We introduced or popularized a lot of dances on our show, including the Twist, although Chubby Checker made it famous. Actually, the kids brought these dances to our shows. I don't know where the kids found them, but they found them fast and came on doing them before I knew about them.

Myself, I don't dance. Naturally. The funny thing is that Mr. and Mrs. Arthur Murray, the famed dance teachers, lived next door to my family in Mount Vernon and gave me free lessons at their studio. I learned how to dance. But the last dance I learned was the Twist. I'm afraid people would expect too much from me, so I pass.

There can be no doubt that eating a balanced diet, skipping the sugary junk foods, staying active, and performing physically in some activity will help you feel, look, and be as young as you can be. A lot of Hollywood stars are running these days. Not only Bruce Dern but Robert Redford, Jack Nicholson, and many others. A lot of them are into tennis. Look what it's done for Charlton Heston and Dinah Shore. But, then, look what it's done for Don Rickles.

I think I get by because I always have been active. I think I would be better off if I were still running or into some specific physical activity beyond swimming, but I don't even like to watch sports, much less compete in them. The most interesting thing I've learned lately is that my beloved pasta, peanut butter, and soft drink are preferable pregame or preactivity foods to steak, salad, and milk because the body digests them better and faster. And a piece of chocolate does provide fast energy, though the lift doesn't last long. But I do keep my weight down, which is important.

I am not a physical fitness nut or a health faddist, but I care about my appearance and my physical condition. I think everyone should care about these things. After all, we not only want to stay young but to live long. I go to my doctor and dentist more often than most people do. I think most people in the public eye do. Maybe we care too much, but we do care. Shouldn't you?

7

Feeling Good

No one dies of old age. We die at different ages. Some people are worn out at forty. Others slow down at sixty. There is no barrier at eighty. We all know people who seem old at fifty and others who seem young at seventy. Many keep going past ninety.

I'm fifty-one and I feel young. I don't feel one day older than when I was thirty. And, as I have said, I am told I don't look one day older. I know I'm older. I've probably lost something. But I don't feel older. And I think a lot of age is in the mind.

If you think old, you'll be old. If the

years scare you, you'll be scared out of years. Once you slow down, it's hard to start up and get back your speed again. What is it that Satchell Paige, the long-lasting pitcher, said? "Don't look back because something may be gaining on you."

No doubt time takes its toll. We die because we wear out. Our bodies break down. Parts stop functioning effectively. We lose strength and the ability to resist disease. But our bodies are like cars. A lot lies in how they're put together. The chemistry has to be good. But it's also a matter of how well we take care of them. Like a finely tuned car, a well-cared-for body will function better and longer.

The major causes of death in the middle years are failures of the heart, lungs, and liver. More than half the deaths in this country result from failures of the cardiovascular systems, which supply blood to the heart, brain, and other parts of the body. Coronary heart disease is the No. 1 killer.

Look it up. I did. Seventy-five years ago heart disease accounted for less than 15 percent of the deaths in the United States. Today that figure is more than 50 percent, partly because of better treatment of other diseases, but also partly because of our softer way of life.

If we stay fit, we'll live longer. It's that simple. If we work hard and rest easy, if we stay active and know when it's time to relax, if we eat right and don't destroy ourselves with drugs, drink, and tobacco, we have a good chance to live to an advanced age and make the most of life as we go.

Unless you get hit by a truck, of course. That's the chance you take every time you cross the street. In California, you may disappear into the ground during an earthquake. Your house may mudslide into the ocean. In New York, you may be mauled by a mugger or starve to death while stranded in a crosstown traffic jam. In Florida, you may be hit by a hurricane. In Texas, by a tornado. In Kansas, by a cyclone. In Louisiana, you may sweat to death. When the wind blows off the lake in midwinter in Chicago, you can freeze to death crossing the street.

I learned long ago not to worry about the things I can't control. I save my worrying for those things I can do something about. I try not to worry about them, I try to do something about them. For most people, survival is a struggle. Times are tough. We have inflation and recession. There's a lot to worry about. But worrying doesn't solve any problems.

I'm not a Christian Scientist, but I do believe our minds control us physically to a great extent. Modern science accepts as fact that excess stress is harmful to us. Clearly, the mind controls a lot of our body. You can't cure a broken leg by positive thinking, but hypertension takes a tremendous toll. Some of us are more resistant to pain than others, though the pain may be the same.

Up to about the age of thirty, the odds are pretty good that you will not have a heart attack. For the next ten years the odds drop to about 30 to 1. For the ten years after that, they are cut in half, to about 15 to 1. For the ten years after that, they'll fall almost by half again, to about 8 to 1. I looked it up. Facts are facts. But the odds are beaten all the time. I feel like I've been beating them. I hope to keep beating them. You can, too.

I was lucky that the drug scene developed after my youth. In my youth, drinking was the thing. It took a heavy toll. And when I got troubled a little later in life, I turned to drink. I am no less subject to such temptations than anyone else. And it almost hurt me a lot. Fortunately for me, I got wise to myself and stopped hard drinking. Clearly, hard drinking is destructive.

Medical science now says a little drinking may be beneficial to the body. A small glass or two of wine, say, is an effective stimulant to the heart. So I follow doctor's advice. Ha! I guess a couple of cans of beer, a couple of glasses of wine, or a couple of cocktails won't hurt most people, but the fact is a little can lead to a lot and the young are right when they say my cocktail-party generation doesn't have the right to put them down for drugs.

Still, drugs are dangerous. Some young people want to live dangerously, but they know how dangerous drugs are as well as anyone. I was just lucky that when the time came to "turn on," I was past that time. Like drink, drugs may make you "forget," but they also will leave you with nothing to remember. I see a lot of people in my business using drugs and I dread the destruction of talent that will follow. I am not even tempted.

Mine did become a generation of pill-poppers. Sleeping pills, stay-awake pills, uppers, downers. Destructive, too. Mind-bending. If you have a healthy outlook on life you don't need such crutches to get through life. The only pills I pop are vitamin pills. I think various vitamins help me. I don't think they hurt me. I've read that pantothenic acid has been shown to prolong life in mammals in laboratory tests. It's one of the B-complex vitamins. These are the only ones with some scientific evidence to suggest they may slow aging. In any event, I take 'em.

I smoked cigarettes for years, but as I said, I stopped years ago. Since the cancer scare, I've seen people stopping all around me. I'm happy to see it. I'm convinced smoking is harmful. It sure can't help you. If you want to stop smoking or drinking and have found it hard, consult your doctor or try a clinic. I'm told many clinics are really helpful to people who want to break bad habits, and I don't see why you should hesitate to try one that is recommended to you by someone who knows. If you feel you need help, seek professional help.

I don't exercise a lot. I should, but I don't. I do a little and I'm determined to do more. I'm going to do some calisthenics. I'm going to ride that damn exercycle. I'm going to swim more. I may even do some running if my feet can take it.

I don't eat right a lot, but I don't overeat. I am active and I do keep my weight down. I think good thoughts. Like about pasta and pretty ladies.

I take care of my teeth. I suffer from periodontitis at times. That's an inflammation of the gums where they meet the teeth. I'm told I'd suffer from it more if I didn't eat a lot of fresh vegetables, raw or undercooked, and other roughage. This helps the salivary glands to wash the teeth. But I eat too many of the sugars that build up bacterial plaque on the teeth, cause cavities, and irritate the gums. My history indicates also that when I worry, it is reflected in my gums. The juices aren't flowing properly or something.

I take care of my body. I do believe that if you take care of your body, it will take care of you. You can't control the chemistry, but you can try to control the things you can control. I get regular checkups from my doctor and dentist, and you should. I have no major health problems, but I want to know about and take care of any problems that turn up. Modern medicine can cure many problems, especially if they're caught in time.

The good doctor Bill Klein, an internist, says, "I consider regular checkups critical to competent health care. Doctors don't practice preventive medicine enough. We tend to treat what we see. But by keeping in close contact with our patients we can at least advise them wisely in advance of probable problems, and catch problems at the outset when they can be effectively treated.

"I separate those people with problems that need constant care and those people with no ongoing problems who appear to be in good health and have no family history of premature heart disease, diabetes, and other things. The American Cancer Society recently recommended that if a person has no known problems he should have a checkup at least every five years up to the age of forty, every two years up to fifty, every year after fifty. I go along with that, but I think after thirty you could do worse than get a check every other year.

"There are physicals and there are physicals, of course. The more complete they are, the better they are. You can't find something if you don't look for it. Of course, a lot of people don't want to know, but it's *not* true that what you don't know won't hurt you. It is the opposite, in fact. What you don't know is apt to hurt you. What you do know you can deal with.

"The more complete the physical, the more costly, of course. It's easy for me to tell you to go all the way. You know what your finances are. But it pays off. Even a complete checkup that does not detect any problems has a positive effect on people, on how they feel, look, and act. Knowing you're healthy is a youthful feeling. It gives you confidence."

What constitutes a "complete" physical? Says Doctor Bill, "I keep a complete history of every patient as a guide to what to look for. In a thorough all-around physical checkup I check everything from weight on. I take different blood tests and urine tests and various X-rays. I check the chest for tuberculosis. I look at the skin. I'm on the lookout for signs of heart trouble, diabetes, and cancer. I make a rectal examination in men, a pelvic examination in women. I think even healthy young women up to thirty should have a Pap smear every two years. Cancer of the cervix is a ten-year-disease. Caught early, it commonly can be dealt with effectively.

"I check for high blood pressure. I

like to take electrocardiograms, though these are not common in routine physicals. I like to know how the heart is behaving beyond what I can hear with my ears. I think treadmill stress tests are desirable periodically. A car may run smoothly while idling, but begin to run rough when subjected to highway speeds. It is the same with the human body. An EKG shows us something. A treadmill stress test, which measures the behavior of the heart when greater demands are made on it, shows more.

"And there are more sophisticated, complex, and revealing tests that show how the blood is getting through the arteries. These tests can be given when a person is known to have, or is suspected of having, heart trouble. Heart attacks, as they are called, of various kinds are not entirely predictable, but if a doctor knows your family history, how you abuse your body and how your body is behaving, he can deal with the probabilities with a fair amount of accuracy. There also are some screening tests that can locate pulmonary problems as they develop and predict their probable development with pretty fair accuracy.

"Thorough physicals by good doctors may cost two hundred dollars or more, but they are really desirable."

How do you find a good doctor? Bill Klein says, "I do not know how you find a good doctor. I think I'm a good doctor, but I'm sure most doctors think they are good. If you're not happy with your doctor, get another one. If you move to a new community, you have to find another one. Your old doctor may recommend a new one, but he can only recommend someone he knows. The local medical society will only recommend several doctors equally. And they only ask their members whether they are willing to take on new patients and in what specialties they consider themselves competent. The doctors do not even have to have board certification, so a medical society recommendation does not guarantee you a good doctor.

"What is a good doctor, anyway? Is he someone who has had special training and board certification in a certain specialty? What type of training? How good a board? Is he a doctor with a good personality or one who listens to you sympathetically? Or is he one with an ability to diagnose accurately and treat properly your problems? I get 75 percent of my patients on referrals from other patients. I guess you have to ask people about their doctors. But there is no guarantee you'll get a good doctor, or even one of the best.

"The general practitioner always has provided, and still provides, the overwhelming share of the primary practice among families. If you have a special problem, your GP will consult with or recommend you go to a specialist. But the general internist is caring for an increasing number of people who want the sophistication of a minimum of two years' residence training in internal medicine. He can provide primary care in a general way, sophisticated care in a specific way; and he can obtain consultations in cases that are complicated beyond the usual. An internist costs more, but I think you may get more for your money. But, there again, a below-average internist is not going to give you as good care as an above-average general practitioner."

Doctor Bill has this to say about staying as young as you can: "No doctor can stop the aging process. There is no pill any of us can prescribe that will keep you young. I am extremely skeptical of any new elixir that is supposed to make miracles. But if you give us a chance, there's a lot a good doctor can do to make you as healthy as you can be and keep you healthy as long as possible. And the healthier you are, the younger you will be biologically.

"Some people look healthy, but they are not. Some people are healthy, but don't look it. What makes one person look young one day and old the next? Appearances are deceiving. Cosmetic surgeons can make you look younger, possibly better, but appearances can be deceiving.

"Life takes its toll of us. The way we feel and look often is reflected not only by what the years have done to us, but by what each day does to us. If you take care of yourself and let a doctor take care of you, you can resist time to some extent," concludes Dr. Klein.

Dr. Lloyd Singer, a fine Huntington Beach, California, dentist, has this to say: "With proper care, your teeth and gums can be kept healthy. Few things make us look as healthy or unhealthy as our teeth and gums. We associate aging with false teeth, for example. Our grandparents lost their teeth one by one. They did not have the benefits of the sophisticated orthodonture we have today, for one thing. Teeth that were crooked often were pulled. They did not have the sophisticated root-canal work that is done today. Abscessed teeth affect the entire body. Teeth that today are repaired and capped were pulled yesterday, and teeth that were pulled were not replaced as well as they are today. Teeth sank in. Cheeks sank in, the nose came down, and the chin came up. Nothing ages a person more.

"The science of capping has been improved enormously. Bridges are built better today. False teeth are made to fit better. Combined with straightening of teeth through orthodontics, these things contribute to a continued youthful appearance in people.

"Naturally, I want patients. But the more regularly I see a patient, the less I have to do to his teeth, the better I can practice preventive medicine or do minor repairs instead of major repairs. I want to do only the work that has to be done. For example, I never recommend capping unless it is necessary to save the tooth or a person convinces me it is critical to him for cosmetic reasons. Ordinary, daily use does some traumatic damage to a tooth and the nerve within. The nerve is the heart of the tooth. The more work we do on a tooth, the more damage we may do to the nerve. If the nerve has had to be removed in root-canal work, then we have to cap the tooth. Otherwise, capping could be too much for the nerve to take. So I try to save the tooth without capping it if I can.

"Regular visits to your dentist will give him the opportunity to practice preventive medicine. For too long now, too many people have been brought up to associate dentists with pain, and so they dread visits to the dentist. Many people do not go to a dentist to have their teeth examined unless they have a toothache or have developed some serious problem. By then they may need large fillings or it may even be too late for fillings and the tooth may have to be extracted. A patient may have to replace his teeth in order to restore his look of youth, the way a plastic surgeon tries to restore a person's look of youth. I think we all prefer the practice of preventive medicine."

Agreed.

8

Face and Other Lifts

People I meet ask me how I stay looking young. It is the question most asked of me. If they've got guts, many then ask if I've had a face-lift. It's the second most-asked question I get. I answer, no, I haven't had a face-lift, but I wouldn't hesitate for a hot minute if I felt I needed one, and I have no doubt the day will come when I will.

I haven't had a nose-bob and I haven't had to have my teeth capped, but I sure don't look down on someone who has. I'd be more apt to look down on someone who needed any of these things and didn't get them done. I don't see why we should be embarrassed or ashamed of doing anything that improves our appearance.

I like looking young. I don't want to start looking older. I will do what I can to delay those days.

My eyesight is still good. At about forty-five I did find I needed reading glasses. I don't need them in my everyday life or for television appearances, so I wear them only when I'm reading. If I need them later, I'll try contact lenses.

Frankly, I think glasses make me look older. I suspect the people who are used to seeing me without glasses would be shocked to see me with glasses and would think I looked older. At least at first. I think if you are used to seeing a person in glasses, they do not necessarily make him look older, but if you are not used to it, and someone starts wearing them, you take it as a sign of advancing age.

I have nothing against glasses. I don't think it's true that men don't make passes at women who wear glasses. I've made a lot of passes at women who wear glasses. My wife is supposed to wear glasses and looks good in glasses, but seldom wears them because she doesn't think she looks good in glasses. I don't think women mind men wearing glasses, and I think many women think men look intellectual and distinguished in glasses.

But if a man doesn't think he looks good in glasses, he should try contacts.

Contact lenses have been improved to the point where they fit well and can be worn comfortably by most people. They can be worn all day and are easy to care for. You can't tell when someone is wearing them. On the other hand, glasses are cheaper and actually enhance the appearance of many people.

Glasses and frames now come in many varied shapes and colors and look very good on many people. For years, women who wear glasses have had several pairs to fit their dress. In recent years, men have started to follow this fashion.

Dr. William Harrison, an outstanding optometrist in Laguna Beach, California, a stylish art colony, provides us with a good deal of practical advice on the matter:

"In the past few years eyeglasses designed for fashion as well as for purely practical purposes have soared in popularity among men following the lead of the ladies. More and more men are getting glasses with a different look for work and for play. They are getting glasses with different-colored frames to suit the clothes they wear on different days. Many men have three or four pairs of glasses ground to the same prescription to suit their various needs.

"Metal frames are sporty, but may not be appropriate for business. Metal frames came into vogue about ten years back and still suit people with small faces very well, but frankly I don't think they suit those with average-size or large faces well, and I think they tend to make a person look older. Personally, I prefer plastic frames of a suitable size and color on most people.

"Plastic frames used to come primarily in solid black or brown, but today they come in various colors of brown, beige, gray, and even blue that will blend in well with a person's skin coloring, his eye coloring, his hair coloring, and the color of his clothes. Black frames are not popular at all. Tortoise-shell frames are not nearly as popular as they were. Many frames come in mixtures of colors that complement a person's coloring and the coloring of his clothes. I like these mixtures. Most are subtle, not bright. Many are neutral enough to fit any color combination.

"If you have dark hair and skin, the basic color of the frame should be dark. If you have light hair and skin, the basic color of the frame should be light. If you have light hair and dark skin or dark hair and light skin, you should use frames of mixed color.

"You should select the shape of your eyeglass frames according to the shape of your face. A person with an angular face will look better with round frames that will soften the lines of the face. A person with a round face will look better with glasses that have more of a rectangular shape that will give his face character.

"One thing most people do not know how to look for is the way the bridge of the glasses is shaped and fits on the nose. If the bridge is longer or fits farther down the nose it shows less of the nose and so makes shorter a nose that may be too long. A bridge that is shorter or fits higher up on the nose shows less of the nose and so makes longer a nose that may be too short.

"I think thinner and lighter frames look and feel better on most people, but if you are a large man and have a large face you can wear a little thicker and heavier frame well. Thinner and lighter frames seem to suit business better than play. Many executives are wearing what are called 'delicatine' frames, which are thinner than the average plastic frames. Coming into fashion now are outsized frames, which, of course, require out-sized lenses and so are expensive. But you'd be right in style with them, as long as you didn't get them too large for your face.

"Also coming into popularity are continuous vision lenses,' which are both practical and stylish. These lenses are ground so that you cannot see the

dividing line or lines separating the varying ground glass a person needs for
bifocals or trifocals. These simply are
more attractive than lenses that are di-
vided and work just as well.

"I prefer plastic lenses to glass lenses.
Plastic lenses can be ground to a
superior optical quality and are not
breakable, as glass lenses are. Plastic is
lighter than glass, so it is especially
suited to the outsized frames. And plastic lenses can be tinted to a variety of
shades for those who wish to have some
color in their everyday glasses, or wish to
avoid glare on their glasses or reflection
off them. The most popular are those
with what is called a 'gradient tint'—
darkest at the top of the grading down to
lightest at the bottom. This color must
match the color of the frame, of course.

"Some people like to wear sunglasses
a lot, and I recommend them for situations in which excessively bright light or
glare will tire or irritate the eyes. But I do
not recommend them for most low-light
situations, those in which the eyes must
strain to see.

"Becoming popular and recommended because they have been enormously improved are sunglass lenses
that change colors, darkening in light
situations, lightening in dark situations.
These are ambermatic or photogray-extra
lenses, and photobrown lenses are being
developed.

"These lenses do pose some problems. The ambermatic tends to a shade of brown in the sun, but to a shade of yellow indoors. This is not attractive and not apt to blend well with the frame or with your skin, unless you're seriously ill. The photogray-extra tends to dark and light gray, which will not match the frames most people want, and, again, hopefully, will not match most skin color. The photobrown-extra may be more attractive when developed.

"Frankly, I believe you should get any sunglasses from an optometrist. Would you buy your regular eyeglasses in a drugstore? If you have a problem that requires prescription glasses other than reading glasses, you should get your sunglasses ground to your prescription. Even if you don't, you want plastic lenses that are prepared properly.

"Many store-bought sunglasses are glass and will shatter. All have molded lenses manufactured on an assembly line and so are of poor optical quality. They will not hurt your eyes in any way, but you are better off with plastic lenses ground to what we call a 50 percent gradient, which is dark enough to be effective in bright light or outdoor situations, but not too dark to be ineffective in low light or most indoor situations.

"The quality of sunglass lenses can be judged just the way you compare a cheap camera and a sophisticated one. It is the quality of the picture that counts. Either you are seeing well what you want to see, or you are not. Cost is not the only consideration. You can pay from $3 up to $40 or $50 in a store for sunglasses, and the price does not reflect the quality of the lens. Nonprescription sunglass lenses are available at an optometrist's for about $35 plus the cost of the frames, while prescription sunglass lenses are $45 to $60 plus frames. The changing color lenses are about $20 more.

"I really believe the extra cost is as worthwhile in sunglasses as in regular glasses.

"Good frames generally range in price from about $40 to $125, with, say, $60 a good average. Single-vision lenses for regular glasses range from $35 to $50. Bifocal lenses cost another $15 or so, trifocal lenses yet another $15 or so. Continuous vision lenses do run $125 or $150 above this. Oversized lenses average about $15 to $20 more than regular-sized lenses. In any event, if you can find a good optometrist, who will take care when making sure your prescription is perfect, you will be getting your money's worth."

Bill Harrison is a good optometrist. He also mentioned an innovation that might be helpful to those of you who have to make speeches or make public appearances, who have to read from notes and are troubled with putting your glasses on and taking them off or troubled with glare reflecting off your glasses and concealing your eyes:

"There is a new type of contact lens system not yet widely known, called 'monovision.' A takeoff on the old monocle, this is a single contact lens, ground to the prescription needed in one eye, usually your worst eye. You wear it as you would any contacts, but only in a specific situation, such as speaking from a prepared text or notes. You can look down and read with one eye, look up, and with your good eye look the audience right in the eyes. You'd be surprised how well it works."

I am not used to myself in glasses, and I think they make me look older. Bill says, "Anyone who is unhappy about his appearance in eyeglasses should try contact lenses. Fitted properly, contacts should not show. And, aside from their cosmetic appeal, they provide superior vision over regular glasses because they sit closer to the eye. In most cases, the stronger a prescription a person needs, the better off he is with contacts. Of course, many people still will need reading glasses.

"Physically, perhaps only 5 percent of the population have special problems, such as misshaped eyeballs, that prohibit the wearing of contact lenses. Another 10 to 15 percent never really feel comfortable in contacts. But, this usually is because people do not give themselves a chance to adjust to contacts, or they have been sold a pair the way a salesman in a store sells you a pair of shoes. You can reshape contact lenses, but you cannot reshape shoes. A good optician will take the time and effort to reshape and readjust your contacts until they are right.

"Almost all discomfort from the wearing of contacts comes from the rubbing of the eyelid on the plastic edges of the lens. The so-called hard lens contacts have 'sharp' edges, and it does take time, perhaps four or five weeks, for the eyelid to adapt to the feel of them. A lot of people do not take this time. The newer, 'soft' lenses have soared in popularity because they are often thinner and do not have sharp edges, so they feel comfortable from the beginning. Also, they are made of a spongelike plexiglass or glasflex, which retains moisture better and is less susceptible to dust. Otherwise, soft lenses are more fragile, harder to care for, and must be replaced more often.

"Because of the way they fit, anyone who is farsighted usually is better off with soft lenses, and anyone who is nearsighted is better off with hard. In general, though, I believe, most people are better off with hard lenses. It has been discovered that the thinner any contact lens is, the better it works, and hard contacts now are being made as thin as soft ones. Surveys show that within four to six weeks, people are as comfortable in hard contacts as soft ones. And the optical quality of hard lenses seems to me to be higher.

"The best lens of all, I believe, is a new silicone lens, which is a hard lens developed in the last year or so and not generally known. It fits comfortably and works really well. All contact lenses can not only correct your vision while being worn but can actually improve your vision. The new silicone lenses so improve many a nearsighted condition that in less than a year, many people with this problem find that even when not wearing the contacts they can see better than they have in years.

"The success of contacts depends on the eye doctor's ability and willingness to adjust the lenses four or five times if necessary over four or five weeks. In many cases it will not take that many adjustments or that long a time, but the optometrist and patient must give it what it takes. The good optometrist uses a good lab that custom-makes each pair of lenses to the patient's prescription, then custom-fits them. You see advertisements offering contact lenses for sale cheap, but what you will get is cheap contact lenses, fresh from an assembly line. Some ads name a price that covers only the cost of the contact lenses and not the cost of the fitting. Any price you pay is roughly half for the lenses and half for the fitting.

"The standard hard lens, fit properly, will run about $200 to $300, depending on the extent of your problem. The soft lens and the silicone lens run about $300 to $350, but the soft lens requires a care kit that cost another $25 to $35.

"If your vision needs correction and you aren't happy in eyeglasses or feel you look older in them, well-ground, well-shaped, and well-fit contacts will help you see better and feel younger, and so you will feel better about yourself and your appearance," concludes the good doctor.

Another thing that can make people look both old and bad are crooked, irregular, or discolored teeth. I've known a surprising number of people who had bad teeth when they were young and not only looked bad because of it but felt bad about it. They hated to open their mouths and often covered their mouths with their hands when they talked. They lacked confidence in their appearance, so their social life was lousy. As soon as they came into some money, they had their teeth fixed. It not only improved their appearance but also gave them a psychological lift. They were "reborn." The cosmetic care of teeth can be critical to good and youthful looks.

Some years back, a lot of parents felt they couldn't afford to have extensive dental work done on their children. When those children grew up, they thought it was too late to have their teeth fixed. Or as they got busy, they didn't want to take the time. Crooked or irregular teeth stayed that way, and because the teeth weren't aligned properly, they often discolored and decayed. Many people have a mouth full of fillings. Nothing makes someone look worse or older. Unless it's missing teeth, obvious bridges, or misfit and dreadful-looking dentures.

I never had to have my teeth straightened. They weren't bad to begin with. I had one tooth pulled early and have a false tooth. I see more and more adults wearing braces these days. They're going in for the orthodontics they were denied or denied themselves earlier. Sure, braces may not look good for a year or so, but when I see people wearing them, I think it's great that they care enough about their appearance to do something about it. The results often are remarkably good. These people look much better and much younger when the work is done. The improvement in their appearance is remarkable.

Many performers have had their front teeth capped. Even ordinary good teeth usually aren't good enough to stand up to the inspection of the close-up camera. It picks up even minor irregularities in the teeth. Capping is not as much trouble as straightening teeth, but it's often more expensive. I doubt that the average person has to have his teeth capped. I'd say more teeth require straightening. But either one can contribute enormously to improved good looks and a more youthful appearance.

Dr. Lloyd Singer, the dentist you met in the previous chapter, says, "More adults are going for teeth-straightening orthodontics than ever before. I guess because more is being made about how people look and more is understood about the benefits. We 'made do' before. We don't have to 'make do' today. The state of the art has advanced, and the results are better. And unlike most things, the price hasn't gone up much, if at all. I don't know why. Maybe because various dental technicians now relieve the dentist of much of the routine work.

"The procedure is generally more difficult with an adult than with a child. An adult's teeth are set, a child's are not. But the results often are equal. For both adults and children, braces are better accepted today than they were yesterday. Years ago, the procedures weren't as perfected as they are today and weren't practiced as regularly. The odd boy who wore braces was considered a "sissy." The rare adult with braces looked weird. But, today, about half our young people get the work done, and the other kids really accept the look. And as more adults are getting into it, it's becoming more accepted. It's sort of a status symbol today. When I see an adult with bad teeth, I think there's someone who doesn't care. When I see an adult with braces, I think, there's someone who cares. And has money." Lloyd laughs.

Lloyd admits that orthodontics can be time-consuming and expensive. "It costs $1,500 to $2,000 on the average and takes eighteen months to two years on the average — often longer for adults. You don't spend a lot of time in the chair, but you do have to go back a lot of times to have the braces tightened and the work checked and changed as needed. With patients who are forty or older, orthodonture is done a lot less for appearance than for performance. But, at any age, the work not only has a good cosmetic effect but a real function. The mouth works better, enabling the teeth to last. Teeth that don't meet, that fail to fit together, don't work well and take a beating in use."

Dr. Singer says, "I do not casually recommend capping. I try to save the tooth first, if at all possible. If you have to have root-canal work, the tooth usually has to be capped. A root canal was all but unheard of not too many years ago, yet it, more than anything else, is responsible for far fewer teeth having to be pulled. The drilling required to clean out a cavity and set the space for a filling does traumatic damage to the nerve.

Capping does additional damage and the nerve sometimes won't survive it. And capping is costly," Lloyd admits.

"But you can guarantee good work in capping teeth more than you can in straightening teeth. Caps are artistically done today and match the shape and color of other caps and other teeth, as they should. You can show the patient just what he's going to get. When it comes to straightening, you can show a patient what you want braces to do, but you can't guarantee the procedure will work perfectly. And you're limited by the position of the teeth and the amount of their irregularity as to how much you can attempt or expect.

"Men and women have different teeth. Within each person's mouth there are many teeth of different shape and color. Matching is critical. You can cap a single tooth in the back of the mouth, but, depending on a person's smile, you usually have to cap two or more teeth in the front of the mouth, or the color and shape will not match as well as they should.

"I do basic dentistry. I cap teeth and I make the molds for the caps, but the caps themselves are prepared at a laboratory. The specialists who make the caps at the laboratory I use are real artists. I think they do the best work of its kind I've ever seen. They do it for the biggest stars in Hollywood. They're located in the Hollywood area. Many dentists who use their work deal with the stars and charge accordingly.

"I happen not to be located in Hollywood or Beverly Hills, but in suburban Orange County, and I charge accordingly. I pay the same amount for the same work from the same lab, but I charge less because my patients usually can afford less. I don't think you can judge the sort of capping you're going to get by the price you're going to be charged, but my price is probably a pretty good average.

"I charge $270 a capped tooth; many Hollywood dentists charge up to $1,000 a tooth. My charge does not vary according to the number of teeth to be capped. If you have two teeth done, it costs $540, and so forth. It is easier to do some teeth than others, and frankly, the cost to me in materials and time to do two teeth close together at the same time is far from double. But I take all that into account when I set the cost per tooth. It is simply easier to set a basic price per tooth."

Dr. Singer also warns that capping teeth takes time: "The time depends on each tooth and the number of teeth to be capped. If they are close together, the dentist can work on several at the same time. If not, you'll need different visits. The teeth have to be drilled down to the stump to which the crown will be attached. Impressions have to be taken so that the crown can be designed properly. The initial visit may last an hour to an hour and a half. Front teeth may take longer because an attractive temporary crown is needed, whereas a less attractive tooth will do in the back. You'll wear temporary crowns while the lab works on the final product. It takes about three weeks to get good caps back from a good lab. It takes about a half hour to install a crown tightly and make sure it fits right.

"Although many of us associate visits to the dentist with discomfort and pain, there really isn't much pain anymore. Pain-killing shots can be given with very little discomfort. There may be some discomfort after a dental procedure, but now it is not usually excessive. Root-canal work has a bad name, but I find the vast majority of patients express surprise at how little discomfort they felt, during and after. There is some discomfort as braces are adjusted. There is some discomfort after extractions, drilling, or drilling down for caps; but with good dentists, it is seldom excessive."

How do you pick a good dentist? Lloyd Singer admits, "I don't know how you select a good dentist, no more than a medical doctor can tell you how to find a good doctor. We'll agree it's important. Even among well-trained dentists, as among well-trained doctors, there's a range in ability from the best to the worst. Some orthodontists straighten teeth better than others. Some specialists do better root-canal work. Some dentists do better fillings. Some cap better than others and use labs that do better work than others. I think the thing to do is to find people who have had the work done that you want done and ask what they thought of the dentist. Then look at the person's teeth and see what you think."

Dr. Singer has this to say about teeth and your appearance: "I don't think many things age a person more surely than bad teeth that haven't been cared for, irregular or discolored teeth, a lot of fillings, missing teeth, badly constructed and installed bridges, poor capping, badly designed and poorly fitting dentures. Few things mar a person's appearance more. And there is simply no excuse for it. If people would take care of their teeth in the first place, they would save them and they would look good. If people haven't taken care of them, their teeth can be repaired. They can be straightened to a great extent. They can be cleaned and filled. They can be capped. And better bridges and dentures can be built.

"I know it can be costly, perhaps uncomfortable for a while, and it does take some time, but you can do something about your teeth, and so to a great extent about your appearance and comfort and health. It just depends on how much you want it. You can save up enough money if you want it enough. Perhaps you can pay in installments. But a lot of your youth lies in your teeth, and if you want to look good, you should have your teeth taken care of." So sums up Dr. Singer.

Plastic surgery, or cosmetic surgery as it is called by the specialists who do it, is less commonly done, seems more extreme, yet sometimes is less expensive than extensive dental work. It also is done now a lot more commonly than it used to be. Nose-bobs, ear-pins, and even face-lifts have become so commonplace that there is little or no embarrassment when someone has one done. And embarrassment is a big part of people's reluctance to have cosmetic surgery.

As more famous people admit to having face-lifts, more people will accept them and be willing to have them done. Beauty is not important to Phyllis Diller's work as a comedienne, for example. Actually, Phyllis isn't bad looking at all. She exaggerates her looks with the wildest getups, makeups, and hairstyles. Yet when she became concerned that her age was showing on her face, she had a face-lift, bragged about it, and made jokes about it. Why not? Why shouldn't she look younger and better? Why shouldn't everyone?

Jolie Gabor, mother of the Gabor sisters, and a great beauty in her own right, threw a party at her Palm Springs home to openly announce her face-lift. And daughters Zsa Zsa and Eva have admitted as much. Few men will admit to a face-lift, as if it's not *macho*, but I don't believe that for a second. I'll have it done when and if I need it.

Few ladies will admit to having had their breasts built up, but some will. More all the time. We worked with a cute little dancer, about eighteen. She had a cute little body, but skinny. Legs up to her chest, and no chest. I thought she looked fine, but I guess she didn't. So she came in one day with cute little breasts bouncing, proud as a peacock of her new look.

If you look in the mirror and you're unhappy with your appearance or with what time has done to you, I think you should do something about it. You may not be able to alter your basic looks greatly, but if you haven't been able to stop what the passage of time and the drift of gravity are doing to you, if you are not happy with what's happening to you and with the toll time is taking, and if you can afford it and it will make you happier with yourself, why not have something done?

There are not many things except cosmetic surgery that can be done for wrinkling, sagging skin. If you have oily skin or if you have taken care to keep your skin well lubricated, you may resist wrinkling and sagging for a long time, or you may never suffer from wrinkling and sagging skin. But most of us eventually will.

There are exercises that help prevent wrinkles. Essentially they consist of making faces, so they probably should be done in private, lest others think you've turned into a raving lunatic. You can do isometrics at your desk, but faceometrics may be frowned on by your fellow workers. Frowned on! Get it?

The face has muscles just like any other part of the body, but we do not exercise our facial muscles as much as we do the others. Exercise strengthens them and helps them hold their elasticity.

With your lips pressed together, smile as broadly as you can and hold that smile for a few seconds. Then relax and repeat this several times. You will find the muscles of your cheeks tensing. Now, open your mouth as wide as you can and hold it open for a few seconds. Relax, then repeat this several times. You will feel the muscles of your cheek, lower chin, and neck tensing.

Open your mouth as wide as possible and close to clenched teeth. Do this again and again in an exaggerated chewing action. You will feel a lot of facial muscles in use. Close your mouth and stretch it from side to side by wiggling your cheek muscles. Wiggle your nose.

Can you wiggle your ears? If you can, you know it is a matter of feeling that muscle just below and in front of each ear and moving it. Those who aren't ear wigglers just haven't found that muscle. The nose muscle is more easily found. If you can feel it, you can move it. Similarly, jaw open, you will feel and can move your neck muscles. Jaw clenched, move your neck muscles.

Open your eyes wide, hold them open, then close them tightly. Repeat this several times. Now raise and lower your eyebrows. Do you feel your forehead moving up and down? Move your forehead muscles. Finally, look in the mirror, make as many funny faces as you can. Some of us can make funnier faces than others. A lot depends on what you're born with.

It's a hell of a way to start or finish your day, anyway.

Exercising the face resists wrinkling and sagging, but once your face has started to wrinkle and sag, it's difficult to conceal.

If you're a lady, you can take a tip from those actresses who wear high-necked and long-sleeved dresses and blouses and wear scarves and things that cover up wrinkled skin and loose flesh, but a man can't do as much of this. In any event, if wrinkled skin or loose flesh bothers you, if your nose or ears or the bags under your eyes bother you, if you feel they make you look older and pose a handicap to you in the pursuit of your profession, you may want to do something drastic about it, such as plastic surgery.

Dr. John Grossman of Denver, a plastic surgeon, says, "I don't think men are looking to regain lost youth in a purely vain sense. I think it has a lot to do with the realization that at the age of fifty or so, when he is still vital and very active, a man may appear to be considerably older. Often he wants to look the way he feels."

Dr. Thomas Rees of New York, says, "When I was training, we were told to beware of men who wanted face-lifts, that they were emotionally unstable. Now our male patients are mainly professionals — lawyers, judges, stockbrokers, clergymen — and they're very stable."

Michael Kamper of Huntington Beach, California, a leading M.D. in plastic and reconstructive surgery, says, "There's a lot that men and women can do to help their appearance and to help them regain the look of youth with cosmetic surgery, and more and more are doing it all the time. As more and more do it, the embarrassment of having had it done becomes less and less. And in many cases no one notices something has been done. The person simply seems to look better. After having had the wrinkles and bags removed from their eyes, many people find their friends simply asking if they are just back from a vacation, saying they look as rested as if they had just been on vacation.

"We can't guarantee that cosmetic surgery won't be noticed. A breast enlargement or reduction on a woman may not be, but a nose-bob or ear-pin or face-lift well may be, especially by people who see you every day. If you would be embarrassed by this, perhaps you will not want this surgery. On the other hand, many are proud of what they've done to improve themselves. I've known many men who pointed out their new noses to friends, as well as women who proudly displayed their 'new' breasts, at least to other women in private."

"Some people have cosmetic plastic surgery because they want to be more attractive to the opposite sex, but many have it simply because they want to be more attractive to themselves. In many cases, the mate is perfectly content with them, but they are not happy with themselves. Many people who are recently widowed or divorced have plastic surgery because they are going back to dating."

The plastic surgeon says, "I find people come to me for cosmetic surgery for many different reasons. It definitely is not only vanity. Many older men come in for surgery that will make them look younger and enable them to better compete in business with younger men. Older men who have lost their jobs will come in for surgery that will make them look younger and give them a better chance of finding new work. Older women who have to work for a living have surgery done to make them look younger and keep them competitive in the marketplace. This is increasing with hard times.

"Young men or women are brought in by their parents for nose jobs, as they are commonly known, or to have their ears pinned back or reshaped. Women come in to have their breasts enhanced or up-lifted, or reduced in size, in some cases. Or tummy-tucks. Men and women come in to have face-lifts, or neck-lifts. Older women come in more commonly for these things, but more and more men are coming in, and more and more age does not matter. At sixteen or sixty, a person needs to be happy about himself or herself."

Doctor Kamper points out that "a good cosmetic surgeon does not tell a patient that work of this sort is going to guarantee getting a job, getting a mate, or even getting a date. Cosmetic surgery is unlikely to make anyone rich and famous. We suggest what they hopefully will look like, but we give no guarantees that it will bring them everything they want out of life.

"A good cosmetic surgeon warns his patients that he cannot predict precisely the exact result of his work. There are too many variables in each person's problem and in the healing process. Some people bring in photos of movie stars and expect to be made into duplicates of these stars. This simply is not possible. We cannot take someone with a thick skin and large-boned nose structure and turn the nose into a tiny, perky nose such as a movie star might have. But we may be able to make a nose look better.

"Before a good cosmetic surgeon proceeds, he makes a judgment on whether or not the prospective patient is not only physically but also psychologically suited for and prepared for the process. If a person can afford it and has realistic expectations of it and can deal with any discomfort that may occur, then we can proceed with the surgery."

The doctor notes: "Cosmetic surgery is surgery, and, basically, all surgery carries with it some risk. The patient has to understand this. There is a very small risk to life. It certainly can't be compared to heart or brain surgery. But there is cutting and there is bleeding and there is some risk. There also always is some risk that the result of cosmetic surgery will leave a patient looking less instead of more attractive than before.

"It is critical to find the most qualified

and skilled surgeon available to you. I
know this is not easy. If you have a doctor, ask him to recommend someone. If
you know someone who has had such
work done, ask this person to make a
recommendation. Most important, make
sure the surgeon has board certification
in the specialty required for a specific
surgery.

"Many doctors, unfortunately, will
say, or even advertise, that they are specialists when they are not. Some say they
are board-certified in cosmetic surgery.
There is no such board. There is a Board
of Plastic and Reconstructive Surgery that
accepts only those who have had special
training and have passed demanding
tests.

"The major libraries have books that
list the special training doctors have had
and the boards to which they belong.
Area medical societies provide this information. Your doctor can obtain it for
you.

"Many have been made happy with
this surgery. It has been of benefit to
many, not only those scarred or de-
formed from some accident, but those
marked by birth or by the years in some
way. And in most cases it is less disabl-
ing surgery and not as costly as many
people think. The advances in the art
have been enormous.

"These days most cosmetic surgery
can be performed in the surgeon's office

instead of at a hospital, and the patient can go home immediately. In many cases, the office operating rooms of plastic surgeons are better equipped and safer for this specialty than those in hospitals. The cost of the office operating rooms is less than that of hospital operating rooms. Hospitals charge by the hour, often $250 an hour for this sort of operation, more if an anesthesiologist is used. Usually, local anesthetic is given in the office and the patient is awake during the procedure, although sedated.

"In many cases, the cost is less than expected, though I do not advise you to shop for bargains. In many cases, the discomfort is less than expected and the recovery period less lengthy. In many cases the results are as expected, sometimes better than expected. As I said, sometimes they are worse. These cases are difficult to predict, and a plastic surgeon who makes promises is to be doubted. None of the cosmetic surgery can be considered simple."

The good doctor specifies: "Nose reconstructions or nose-bobs as they are commonly called, used to be the most common cosmetic surgery. Yet they are the most difficult to do. And the results are the most difficult to predict. All noses are drastically different, so all nose-bobs are drastically different.

"Because outside scars on noses are impossible to hide, we work on the inside of the nose. The bones are broken with a small mallet and a chisel. Some of the bone is frequently chiseled away. The bone is then reset in the desired shape. We depend on the skin to shrink down to fit the new bony framework underneath during the healing process. This does not always happen as we want it to. Often it does, and the nose assumes the desired shape.

"If the surgeon has his own operating room in his office, this is where the nose-bob is done. The average cost for routine work of this kind is about $1,500, plus about $200 for the operating-room fee. If done in a hospital, the additional cost is about $500. The surgical fee can vary widely, depending on many factors, including the area where the doctor's office is located. It takes one and a half to two hours to do this surgery."

When it comes to pain, the doctor says, "There will be less discomfort than you might expect. With your nose packed, you will have to breathe through your mouth. Many find this uncomfortable. You will have 'black eyes' and other facial discoloration. Within a few weeks, this will pass. In about two weeks you will be able to go back to light work and in about four weeks you will be able to go back to heavy work.

"Nose-bobs are not as common as they once were. I don't know if you can attribute this to the natural look being favored by the young now, to the popularity of Barbra Streisand and her nose or others. Conversely, there are more of the other cosmetic operations being done than before. There are more breast enhancement operations being done now in cosmetic surgery than any other kind. Some women also are having 'tummy-tucks' done so they will look better in bikinis. Skin stretched through pregnancy or the carrying of excess weight is tightened.

"Ear-pins are rather common cosmetic surgery for both sexes. A lot of people feel their appearance is hurt by ears that stick out. A lot of parents have this surgery done on their children, who often are kidded about 'Dumbo ears' by other kids. This operation can be done from about the age of six on. I worked on one man who was fifty. He had always wanted it done and felt he finally could afford it.

"An ear-pin operation can be done in the doctor's office or at a hospital. It costs $1,000 to $1,250, plus the cost of the operating room. The protruding ears simply are pulled back with inside stitching. It takes two to two and a half hours to do this. The patient must wear a head bandage for about one week and avoid excessive exercise for about four weeks."

As for face-lifts, our expert says these are second only to nose reconstructions in difficulty: "The surgery does vary widely, depending largely on whether specific work in the area of the neck or the eyes is critical to the basic operation. The degree of predictability varies. Each procedure can be done separately, but sometimes all are covered in a single surgery.

"All can be done in office operating rooms. The patient does suffer more discomfort from face-lifts than from some other cosmetic surgery, and the recovery period is longer. There will be discoloration, swelling, and soreness, which will last two to three weeks or so. The operation runs four hours or so, and having the operation done in a hospital increases the cost.

"Basically, we cut the skin where it is least likely to show when it heals, such as inside the hairline and around the ear. We separate the skin from that which is beneath it, pull it up, cut off the excess, and sew it up. This usually takes care of sagging jowls and the so-called turkey neck. Basically it smooths the wrinkles age puts on our faces. The hanging overskin, or bags, which develop beneath the eyes are dealt with similarly but separately. We do not pull too tightly for fear of giving the face the look of a mask. Skin that is too tight looks unnatural. We want to retain some expression lines and so retain the character of the face.

"The average cost of a face-lift is about $2,000 to $3,000, plus $300 or so for the office operating room. Here again, hospitals charge considerably more, perhaps $1,000 more. Eyelid work runs from $1,000 to $1,800, plus $200 to $300 for the office operating room. Again the hospital cost will add $500 or more."

For the information of men whose women may be interested in breast enlargements or reductions, or for the women who may be reading this, the good doctor provides some details: "Aside from providing replacement breasts after mastectomies, we do a lot of work on young women who want their breasts enlarged and some work on those who want them reduced. Being oversized may pose as many psychological problems as being undersized. And many women come to me in their forties or fifties. Certainly these women have many years left to live and are entitled to look as good as they can.

"Breast enhancement operations are less difficult to do than breast reduction operations. Breast enhancement operations can be done in an office operating room, but reductions must be done in the hospital. Implanting silicone bags beneath the breast takes two or two and a half hours; breast reductions take about twice as long. Breast enhancements cause less discomfort. The recovery period is three to four weeks. Breast enhancements cost between $1,500 and $2,000 on the average, plus

about $250 for operating room costs —
another $400 or more in the hospitals.
Breast reductions may run $1,000 or so
more."

Concludes the cosmetic surgeon: "We
can't stop the clock. We can turn it back
a little sometimes. We can turn it back
more than once, as by doing more than
one face-life. We can't guarantee to make
you look twenty years younger or ten
years younger or five years, six months,
and seven days younger, but we can frequently make you look younger. We frequently can make you look better. How
much younger and how much better depends on many factors. Whether you
want to look younger or better badly
enough to have such surgery depends on
you."

As I see it, an increasing number of
people seem to want cosmetic surgery,
and I see no sin in it. To a great degree,
we are what we seem to be. If we look
old, we are old. If we look bad, we are
unattractive. I don't care if you are going
after a job or a mate, you will be best off
when you look your best.

9

Sex and the Younger Mate

like young women. I like sex. I like young girls, too, but fortunately I do not think of them sexually. Teen-agers do not turn me on sexually. If they did, I'd be in deep trouble because I've worked with them on the "Bandstand" show a long time. I was important to some of them, and I'm sure I could have had some of them for the asking. I never asked. A few threw themselves at me. Sadly, they had to be thrown off the show. Many people in my business, disc jockeys and the like, who deal with young girls, have not been able to resist temptation. A couple have been caught

and disgraced. I've never been more than
mildly tempted and have not been soiled
by that sort of scandal.

I do like young women. In my teens
and twenties I went out with girls my
own age. In my thirties I went out with
young women in their twenties. In my
forties I often went out with women in
their thirties. I did not cheat on my
wives, but I dated between my marriages.
Each of the three marriages I have made
has been to a woman who was progres-
sively younger than I was. My first marriage was to a woman one year younger,
my second to one six years younger, my
third to one thirteen years younger. Is
this a weakness in me? I hope not. I
think not. Many of us are attracted to
younger mates. Others are attracted to
older mates. It's something in our personalities, I suppose.

It's always been more common to see
older men with younger women than
older women with younger men. So it's
become more accepted. But it's almost
always assumed that the old guy feels
flattered by the attention of the young gal
and is willing to look like a fool to gain
her favor, in or out of bed. It's almost always assumed the young gal is willing to
sacrifice sex, to let the old geezer get his
hands on her in order to get her hands
on his money. Provided he has money, of
course. Often, the older guy has gained a

place in life that the younger guy is just going for.

All these assumptions are often true. You seldom see a well-off guy with a homely gal. Unless he married her when he was young and poor. If so, he sometimes divorces her and takes up with a younger, more attractive gal after he makes his fortune. And if a guy has money, he usually has a wide choice and picks from among the pretty ladies interested in him and his money. Anyone with a choice — star athletes, screen stars, and such — almost always picks a pretty lady. Which often is unfortunate. If a gal is both attractive and pleasant, great. But in the long run, the pleasantness, the intelligence, all the things that matter in a person, are more important than the prettiness.

Luckily, it is not true that a man always picks a lady for her looks, anymore than it's true that a woman always picks a man for his looks. It's often not true that a younger lady picks an older man for his money, or an older man picks a younger lady for her sex or to enlarge his ego. There are many things that attract one person to another, and we have to stop making assumptions about these situations. I think many have stopped making these assumptions.

For example, it's almost always assumed that when an older woman takes up with a younger man, she is on an ego trip and trying to recapture her lost youth and trying to prove that she is still sexually attractive. I suppose this has been true many times. But I'm also sure it's not true many times. Today, older women are seen with younger men more and more. And so it is beginning to be better accepted. And the assumptions are beginning to disappear.

Obviously, wherever you have a younger person with an older person, you also have an older person with a younger person. I don't think there's anything wrong about this, either. I think society is starting to accept the fact that age is far from the only thing and nowhere near the most important thing in picking a partner. I really don't think we should worry about what society thinks, anyway. No one really knows what's going on in another person's head. Often, even the person isn't sure. No one really knows what's going on between two people. They're the only ones who know anything about it. I try not to judge other people or other marriages. When I do, I'm often wrong. No one knows what goes on behind closed doors.

An older person may seek a return to youth through a younger mate. An older person may feel younger by dating the sort of young person he dated when young. An older person may be seeking the energy and curiosity and perhaps even innocence that often can be found in a younger partner. On the other hand, a younger person may be seeking the experience and knowledge and insights that frequently can be found in an older partner. A younger person may feel more mature by association with an older person. A younger person may feel more settled down with an older person.

I'm an old guy who likes young gals. I'm not truly old yet. I don't feel old. I don't look old. I try not to think old. I look young and I'm trying to stay young. That's a big part of this book: staying young. I have to assume that if you're reading this book, this is something you're interested in, too. So, while I see nothing whatsoever wrong with seeking older mates, I want to talk here about seeking younger mates and how I think it helps a person to stay young.

When you take up with a younger person, you are pulled into her more youthful world. If you're going to keep up with that person, if you are going to keep the connection, you are going to have to understand your new mate's world, which may be as new to you as if you never were there yourself. You never were. That was another world you were in when you were young.

Of course, the other person is pulled into your world, too, and also has adjustments to make if he or she is going to make the relationship work. But in this book I'm interested in the way an older person can stay young by associating with young people and often by going to a young mate.

I absolutely am not advocating you throw over your old mate. If you are happy with your mate, great! There are a lot of ways to recapture youth or stay young. Finding a young mate is only one way, and it's not necessarily the best way. But, if you are free, it is one way and can be a good way.

My first marriage was to Barbara Mallery. I met her in high school in suburban New York when I was fifteen and she was fourteen. I had acne and I was shy with girls. I hadn't dated much, didn't have much experience with girls, and so wasn't totally comfortable around them. But I was interested in them. I was a normal, red-blooded lad who looked at girls and thought of sex. Barbara was a beautiful, blue-eyed brunette. She was a cheerleader, rah-rah. A buddy of mine was dating her, and he arranged a blind date for me so that we could double-date. At the last minute my date got sick. My buddy and Bobbie insisted I go along with them anyway. We went to the movies and, afterward, to the soda shop. I was smitten.

Soon I was the one dating Bobbie, and before long we were going steady. We went together hot and heavy for a time. Frankly, it was so hot and heavy we decided to cool it for a while. We spent a winter apart, dating others. Then chance threw us together again, and the old spark caught fire again. We started going steady again and continued through my high school graduation.

Her family moved to Maryland, and mine moved to upstate New York. While I was starting college in Syracuse, she was finishing high school in Salisbury. This was thirty years ago, and I made many a round trip, seventeen hours each way, in a sixteen-year-old convertible. There was no heater and the winter trips, even bundled up, were really Frosty the Snowman.

I dated other girls at Syracuse, but I regarded Bobbie as my girl. She spent one year at a state teacher's college in Maryland, then was allowed to transfer to another one in Oswego, near Syracuse. We spent our weekends together, going to movies and dances, drinking beer with my buddies from my frat house, stealing sex whenever we could. I "pinned" her, then gave her an engagement ring I got at a bargain from a buddy's jeweler father. We decided to wait a year to be married, until she graduated and I had gotten a start in the outside world.

The funny thing is, I don't even remember asking her to marry me. Or even her asking me. It was sort of assumed by our families and friends, and by us, too.

By that time we had gone together so long that we just sort of drifted into marriage. We were used to each other and comfortable with each other.

While I was working in Utica, I was making out at times with an occasional girl in the back seat of my car. I think the passion had paled by the time I went to Maryland and married Bobbie in June of 1952. I was started in Philadelphia by then and brought her back there with me. We found an apartment in the suburbs. A son, Richard, was born in January 1957.

I was busy working, making my show work, making my fame and fortune. Bobbie taught for a while, then quit to take care of our son. She wasn't swept up by show business and stayed home a lot. We moved into three different apartments — in one of which we appeared with Edward R. Murrow on "Person to Person." He interviewed us from his studio. Later we bought a house. I wasn't home a lot and neglected Bobbie a lot.

When I said earlier that our marriage ended when a friend called up to tell me her husband was running around with my wife, that was simplification at its most unfair. Our marriage might have been saved, but there was nothing to save. I had stopped telling my wife I loved her, and she had told me she felt she had never really loved me, which hurt a lot. We talked it over and decided to divorce. When we separated, Dickie went with her, which hurt, too. Our divorce was granted in November of 1961, so our marriage lasted a little less than ten years.

In 1959 I put together *Dick Clark's Caravan of Stars* and started to take tours with it. The tours were remarkably successful; we frequently did $5 million worth of business a year. One of the singers on a tour in 1961 was Joanne Campbell. Her secretary, Loretta Martin, traveled with her. So she also traveled with me. This was during my divorce. I was depressed and lonely. Friends say I was bouncing back from a busted marriage in the usual way, but I met Loretta, started to date her, and felt like I had really fallen for her.

She was pretty, tiny, brown-eyed, blond. About five feet tall and full of life. It turned out to be very easy for her to get full of life. We married in April of 1962. Our first child and my second, Duane, was born in March of 1963, and our second and my third, Cindy, in January of 1965. The kids became my wife's whole life. I love my kids, but my life included other things.

I don't think there is a right or wrong in these things. I went into marriage with a traditional view of it. I figured you found a lady, loved her, married her, had kids, had a house, and a "normal life," till

death did you part. But the show business life I landed in wasn't normal. I
worked hard. I was ambitious, busy. I
wasn't ready to settle down. Maybe I
never really will be.

Maybe I went into marriage for the
wrong reasons. I was disappointed that
my first marriage didn't work and was
anxious to prove I could make a marriage
work. But I wasn't ready to work at it. I
was lonely and wanted to be loved, but
not ready to give to a marriage what it
needed.

In any event, my second marriage
didn't work almost from the start. We
went into it too soon and didn't know
each other well enough. She fell for me,
too, and maybe expected more from me
than she got. I know now that you have
to give a lot to a marriage.

We argued. We tried to talk it out. We
tried to make it work. We tried for three
or four years. We really tried. But if feelings aren't there the way they should be,
if the chemistry is wrong, you can't make
a wrong marriage right.

I remember telling Bobby Darin that
Loretta and I had decided to end our
marriage. I said I hated the thought of it.
He said that if something wasn't working
out, it was wise to end it. He was right.
Loretta and I were hurting each other
and beginning to hurt the kids, who were
young and impressionable. Loretta and I
separated in 1970. We knew we couldn't

pick up the pieces, but we didn't rush out and get divorced. Both of us were soured on marriage by then and disappointed in ourselves.

We found we could be friends, if not mates. Once the friction of two ill-suited people rubbing on each other in everyday life ended, we found we could talk to each other and understand each other's problems.

Bobbie and I also are friendly. After our divorce Bobbie remarried and moved to Ohio. While I did not get to see my son as much as I would have liked, I got to see him in summers and usually had three full months with him.

Loretta has not remarried and has stayed in Southern California, and so I get to see a lot of our son and daughter. They are still in school.

I see a lot of my oldest son now. He's working out here, interested in show business, trying to figure out exactly what he wants to do in the business. I tell him to try everything, to open himself to experience, and to go after it hard when he finds out what "it" is.

Fortunately, my three kids have managed to handle their parents' divorces well. They're all bright, attractive, healthy and active. They spend many hours with me these days, and I'm really proud of them.

I met Karen Wigton in our offices. Everyone calls her Kari. She was working in accounting. She grew up in a small town in Minnesota. Her father owned a bar, while her mother was a schoolteacher. Her mother never had a drink in her life. It was a funny combination, but it worked. They had a happy marriage and a happy family of four. They made Kari happy. She went to North Dakota State University and the University of Oregon, studying speech and dance, but she never went into performing. Instead, she went to work in Washington, D.C.

She worked for Senator Quentin Burdick of North Dakota and Representative Wayne Hays of Ohio. Yes, Wayne Hays. Kari swears she never had a personal relationship with the colorful congressman. She took a leave of absence to go on a "Discover America" tour. For a year she visited interesting cities around the country. The last city, Los Angeles, really got to her. She never left. She got a job in my office.

I liked her right off. My marriage to Loretta was over. Since I didn't have a warm, personal relationship in the last years of my marriage, I was hungry for one. Kari gave me a lot of love. Almost as soon as we started to date, we started to go together constantly. Instead of asking her to marry me, I asked her to move in with me. She was willing. She understood me. Always has. I'd had two bad marriages and was scared of a third. I felt like a two-time loser. Like I had a police record. At first I didn't even seek a divorce, as if doing so would free me to commit another crime. I'm not "Hollywood" to the extent I can take marriage and divorce in stride as part of a package.

Kari didn't care that I'd had two marriages before and that neither one had worked. She wasn't my other wives, she was who she was. I was who I was. What was between us was different from what was between any other two people. What didn't work with others might work with us. Living together was the new thing to do. One of the things I got from Kari was a willingness to try new things. Another thing I got from her was a willingness to try a new marriage. You don't give up on good things. A good marriage can be great. We found living together was great. We got along great. We got a lot out of life. She brought a whole lot of youthful enthusiasm back into my life.

I got my divorce in December of 1975. Even so, Kari and I didn't rush into marriage. We had lived together seven years before we married on July 7, 1977. It turned out to be the lucky number to beat all lucky numbers, 7-7-77. I hope it turns out to be good luck for us. I feel it was lucky for me. Put together the seven years we lived together and the three we've been married and we've made it to ten years and beaten the real life span of my two previous partnerships with the opposite sex.

Kari is twelve years younger than I am, but that doesn't matter to me. I don't think it matters to her. But I suppose I should let her speak for herself:

Kari Wigton Clark says, "The difference in our ages never mattered to me. Dick seemed young to me and still does. He looks young and acts young. He stays young in the way he dresses and talks and thinks. I suppose I give him some of my youth, but he gives me some of his. I think what I gave him more than anything was an added incentive to do well and live life to its fullest. A new relationship can do that for someone. He gave me new incentive. I'm very adventurous and he added a lot of adventure to my life. He lets me find new vacation places, and he's ready to go. I have some interests that are different from his, but he's become interested in my interests. That's the way he is. I've taken an interest in his interests. That's the way we both are.

"When I went into this thing, I just thought of it as an affair. I figured as long as it lasted, fine. I hadn't been married and wasn't bent on being married. I knew he'd had bad marriages, if it's fair to call them that, and I was happy just to be living with him. But our life together was so good, we decided to put it on a permanent basis. I never gave a second thought to his other marriages. I didn't know about them, but I knew about him. My head was on straight. We'd lived together a long time, and we knew we were compatible. Actually, what it is, I'm compatible. He's not. I make us compatible. He's moody, up and down, but I'm always in a good mood, always up. He's got a good thing going, and I won't let him forget it or give up on it if I can help it."

So concludes Kari. I guess we're lucky to have each other. Such perfect people! Actually, she's right. I do ride a roller-coaster of emotions. It's the nature of my work. Up and down. Exciting. Love it. It keeps me young. But she keeps me in my place. When I get too high, she brings me back to earth. When I get down in the dumps, she lifts me up. She is even-tempered and level-headed. And our relationship did refresh my interest in life. I don't know about the new interests she brought me. She's interested in dogs. Two dumb dogs is what she brought me. And a new lust for love. I like the dogs. I love the lady. And love making love to the lady.

Despite my experience with vitamin E, I really don't think there's any drug that can increase your sexual potency. I think it's in the mind. Sex is a state of mind. Some of us think of it more than others, and some want it more than others. I don't say you have to be an

animal about it, but I suspect the more
you want it, the more youthful you are.
Those that drop out of the sex scene
tend to feel older, over the hill.

I believe it's important to have a partner who is compatible with you in most
ways, including sex. If the chemistry is
right between you, you will overlook a lot
of the other's faults and overcome a lot of
obstacles. But if the sexual chemistry is
not right, it causes a constant tension
and builds a barrier between the two of
you that you may not be able to get over.
The partner who is not wanted will feel
unloved, undesired. The older partner
who is not wanted will feel washed up.
He or she certainly will not feel good
about himself or herself.

If you're lucky enough to have a partner who is suited to you sexually, you've
got a lot going for you. You do have to be
lucky. Some of you no doubt do not have
partners with whom you're compatible
or perhaps do not have sexual partners
at all. A lot of things I've written about in
this book will help you find a suitable
partner. If you're looking good and staying young, you will be more attractive to
the opposite sex. If you feel good about
yourself, if you feel young, you will have
confidence and will act accordingly. A
person who looks good, who seems
youthful, who acts with confidence, is attractive to others.

I know that when I'm overweight I

feel lethargic. When I'm thin, I feel energetic. When I feel good about myself, I'm interested in sex. I think Kari feels good about herself because she's usually interested in sex. When I want it, she seems to want it. When she wants it, I usually want it. To a great extent, being wanted turns you on. And desire turns off tiredness. It's amazing how fast you forget how tired you are when you get turned on.

I can't always have Kari when I want her, nor can she have me. She works with me, and there is no way I am going to throw her on a desk in my office in the middle of a workday and have my way with her. There's a constant stream of workers and visitors through our offices, and neither of us is an exhibitionist. Also, I suspect it would be bad for business. Occasionally she tries to throw me on a desk, but I fight her off. I am a man of high principles.

Yet, there are times when our eyes meet, when we touch, when we know what's ahead. All couples know this feeling. And it's a fine feeling. It's a comfortable feeling. Anticipation whets the appetite. I can concentrate on other things in the meantime.

I don't think Kari minds my talking about us like this. I don't think we're unique. I hope not. We've got a good thing going. I hope we can keep it going. I hope there are a lot of you out there with this sort of thing going, and I assume there are.

One of the things Kari has brought to me, one of the youthful things, is a wonderful openness about sex. We not only have it when it's reasonable to have it, but we kid about it, talk about it, and are not ashamed about it. It's the most natural instinct on earth, yet for years people, even married people, weren't supposed to talk about sex in public. It was as if they weren't doing it, as if it were a shameful thing to do. More and more, sex is admitted, accepted. Sex has come out of the closet. Or bedroom. And it's beautiful.

Young people are open about sex. They admit to it. "Admit" isn't the right word. And they don't "brag" about it anymore. "Brag" isn't the right word. The word is "accept." Young people accept sex. Married or not. In the dating situation. Earlier than ever.

I'm not sure all of this is good. Casual sex can have bad results. Not only unwanted pregnancies and, maybe, abortions, but disappointment in sex and a loss of love. I think a very real, good feeling for the other person should go with sex if sex is going to work well for you. But I do think it's good that we can accept sex openly as a part of life and that we are not ashamed of it. If we feel ashamed of it, we shouldn't have it.

If you have the right partner, you will

be able to be open about sex, and you will be able to satisfy each other. You will not have to hint around, wondering how to approach your partner. Asked, you can say yes or no, openly. Hopefully, you will not say no too often. Too many no's build barriers. You won't both feel like it at the same time every time. But it is best to respond to your partner in some way. It is important to make your partner feel good about herself or himself, and usually this will make you feel good about yourself.

There are a lot of ways. As a prelude, try a sensual massage. Use a massage lotion to lubricate the skin. This is one cosmetic type of treatment that requires a partner. In this case your partner's loving attention is obviously another aid to help you feel young! Doing it different ways is in itself a youthful thing. It makes the act new and fresh, and there is a sense of discovery. It brings you two a feeling of intimacy. And a sense of sharing that strengthens the bond between you.

Usually one of you will want it more. If you're a good match, you can compromise. If once a month satisfies you, OK. It's your bag. If once a week, fine. I don't think we should put sex on a schedule, like every Saturday night after the bath. If you want it all the time, great. You ought to be doing it every five minutes. As far as I know, there's no rule.

Get rid of any restrictions you feel. They're not there if you don't put them there. The new thing is to accept sex as an important part of life. The youthful thing is to be open about sex and enjoy it.

Keep yourself looking good, and your sex life should be doing good. Keep yourself clean, neat, and looking as young as you can, and you will feel young and want sex. And you will get sex and get pleasure from it and give pleasure in it. You may not be able to perform with all the acrobatics of your younger days, but you will be able to perform. Sex will make you feel young, and it will help you stay young.

10

Eternal Youth

There is a fountain of youth, and you can drink from it. I found it, and so can you. It is not something you'll find somewhere, like a gurgling piece of sculpture in a plaza in Florida. It is in your head. Use your head, and you can keep or rediscover your youth.

Don't worry about the things you can't control. Do something about the things you can do something about.

Take care of yourself. Take care of your body. Take care of your health. Exercise adequately and eat intelligently. Slim down and get in shape. Get regular checkups from your doctor and dentist.

Deal with any physical problems you have.

Clean up and straighten up. Take care of your skin. Take care of your teeth. Take care of your hair. Stand tall and take the world in. See what's going on around you. Be conscious of styles. Dress in fashion. Wear your hair in fashion. Be neat and well-brushed and well-dressed and in step with the times. Get with the world the way it is, not the way it was.

If it takes drastic measures to make yourself the way you want to be, do whatever you can do, have done whatever can be done. If baldness bothers you, get a hairpiece. If you don't like your nose, a bob may make it better. If you don't like the lines on your face, get a face-lift. If plastic surgery may give you a lift, give it a chance.

So people didn't do some of these things yesterday. They're being done today. You have to look at life from fresh perspectives. You may have to keep an open mind. Tomorrow will bring more new things. Talk to people who've done new things, different from the things you do. Look into any activity that interests you. Don't live in your yesterdays. Take each day as it comes. Make the most of today. And look forward to your tomorrows.

Keep up with the times. As the times change, the world changes. Change with it. Don't be afraid to rethink your thinking. Don't be afraid to turn an open mind on to new ideas. Don't be afraid to alter your values. Don't be afraid.

With each birth, I think the world is reborn. Every new person sees a new world in a new way. Each generation takes what has been left to it and builds a new world on it. The young break down old barriers and set out in new directions.

Personally, I think the young are responsible for most progress.

All progress is not good. Overpopulation crowds cities and consumes our resources. As money decreases in value, unemployment increases. And crime increases. But I do believe we've made tremendous progress in our personal freedoms.

We've dropped a lot of our old hangups. We look at life as it is and don't have to dread telling it as it is. Minorities are beginning to be accepted in all walks of life the way they should have been many years ago. The women's movement is giving women the equality with men they should have had all along. With it, relationships between men and women have become better, more realistic and honest.

I credit the kids for this to a great extent. I think we should let them into our lives and look at their way of life and take from it what will help us live our lives better.

We should talk to our children, talk to

young people, listen to what they have to say, try to understand them. We should not only give them what we have to give but take from them what they have to give. Youth is a contagious condition. If we take youth from youth, we can give others around us some of this youth.

We should welcome youth into our lives. We should welcome young ideas into our oldest attitudes. We should welcome young ideas in our corporations. We should try to plan our play and our work with the enthusiasm, energy, and imagination of youth.

I do not make New Year's resolutions, but every year or so I sit down with myself and look at where I've been, try to figure out where I'm at, and decide where I want to go. I take a hard look at the old things I'm doing to see if they're still working, and take a long look at new things I might do to see if they can be made to work.

I'm in a couple of comfortable ruts, but I rouse myself regularly by doing some daring things simply because I think we all have to keep setting new goals for ourselves to make ourselves reach as far as possible. I relish challenge. Few things that are easy to do are worthwhile. Doing difficult things can be enormously satisfying.

Embark on new adventures as often as possible. Approach each adventure with the intensity of youth. You haven't done everything yet. You may have succeeded at some things, but there are other things to try. You may have failed at some things, but there are other things to try. You're not dead, so you're not defeated.

New projects give me get-up-and-go and keep me feeling young. I wake up every morning looking forward to the day. I know I'm going to have problems. I have 'em every day. I know some things won't work. I know there'll be frustrations and disappointments. But I do not give up easily, and I look forward to overcoming obstacles. I love my work.

If you are not happy in your work, get into another line of work. I don't care if you're successful or not. I don't care if you're making a lot of money or not. If you're not happy, what good is the rest of it? If there's something you always wanted to do, do it. Find something you want to do. Start again if you have to. Take a cut in pay. But take a chance.

Gauguin gave up banking to become a painter. I don't know if he found happiness, but he gave the world some great art. Doing what he wanted to do must have given him some happiness. I guess he had to give up his family, but to him it was worth it.

You hear every day of people who have given up professions to sail around the world. It takes courage. I admire this kind of courage. Maybe it won't work.

What the heck, whatever the person was doing before obviously wasn't working for him, either. At least he or she is trying, going for the brass ring.

Garage mechanics quit to breed dogs. An old guy or gal goes back to college to pursue a new course, perhaps one they always wanted. I say, buy a boat, breed a dog, get a degree.

Make the most of your work. Look at it the way you did when you were just starting out. Make a new start. And if your present work isn't satisfying you, make a new start in another direction. We aren't capable of doing all things, but we all have different things we can do. We all should be the best we can be. If you have a family, level with them. Tell them if you're unhappy, and tell them what might make you happy. Try to get them to go along with you.

I'll never retire because that would be like saying my day was done. But if you think differently and are retired, look for a job, seek a hobby that will make you happy, find something to do with your days that will make them full. If you're married, look for things to do that will fill your relationship, rekindle the old flame. Have sex at high noon. Take off on impulse on a trip.

There's nothing better than a good marriage and nothing worse than a bad marriage. The same applies to any relationship. If you've got a good relationship, treasure it. If you've got a bad one, end it. Seek a new one. Seek one in which you can be happy. And in which you can make someone else happy.

I hated to see my first two marriages break up. I felt I had success in my professional projects and failures in my personal relationships. But I knew it was wise to let my marriages go because they weren't going anywhere. I think my former wives are happier, and I know I'm happier. I could see that as traumatic as it was on the kids to break up the families, children are better off being brought up in homes that are not torn apart by arguments and darkened by anger and depression.

I never gave up my kids. They have lived with their mothers, but I have spent as much time with them as possible. I always have let them know they have a father who cares about them, and they know I am always available to help them. I would have preferred to have been a closer part of their daily lives, but it wasn't possible. You have to take life as it is.

I am glad I did not give up on marriage. I have found a mate who makes me happy, who seems to be made happy by me. She is younger than I am, but that doesn't matter. Not the difference in age. I borrow on her youthful confidence, curiosity, and vitality and try to repay her with interest with my dedication to life and to staying young. With her, I am enjoying my life more now than ever before. For her, I want to be successful, not only at work but in life. We want this marriage to work. To work, we have to keep it alive.

We share everything in our lives. Unless you can share them, the successes don't amount to much and the failures are almost too much to bear. We try to be open with each other in all aspects of our lives. If you don't have someone with whom you can share the stuff of life and with whom you can be intimate and open, look for someone else. Even the seeking can be satisfying. At least you are looking. You're off your rear end, up on your feet, and on the move.

Many have had less success, more failures, and much greater tragedies in their lives than I have. But I have learned that success is frequently elusive, failure frequently inevitable. It is the going on, the bouncing back, the fresh beginnings as if we were young again that matter most and give meaning to our lives. Tragedies sometimes have to be borne.

Above all, we have to be happy with ourselves. Different people find happiness in different ways, but we have to look for it for ourselves. We have to take pride in ourselves, pride in our appearance, pride in our attitude, pride in our performance. I will never give up going for success in my professional life and my personal relationships.

We do not have eternal youth, but we can live our lives as if we do. There is a lot to be said for the phrases, "young at heart" and "young in spirit." The years take their toll, but we can steal time if we try; we can reduce our losses. We can't live forever, but we can make the most of the years. We can live with youthful enthusiasm and energy. We can do our best to stay young, look good, and enjoy life.

There is nothing wrong with being fifty. Or being thirty or forty or sixty or seventy. I am not ashamed to admit I'm over fifty. Frankly, I wish I were twenty, but there you are. I don't want to pretend I'm twenty. Or even thirty. And I wouldn't want to give up what I've gained with the years. With experience, we learn a lot — if we're interested in learning. I'm interested. And I'm learning every day.

I'm fifty-one. I'm happy to be there. As they say, the alternative is a lot worse! But I'm also happy I look young for my age. I want to look good. I want to look young. I want to think young. I want to be as young as I can be until the day I die. I don't want to look or think or act any older than I have to be. And that's the way I think you should be. And can be.

ABOUT THE AUTHOR

Long one of America's favorite entertainers, Dick Clark is regarded as the personification of perpetual youth. Not a day passes that someone doesn't come up to him and ask, "How do you stay so young? What's your secret?" Thinking young and staying active are certainly part of the answer.

Born on November 30, 1929, in Mt. Vernon, New York, Dick Clark became fascinated with "the magic world of radio" while attending high school. During 1947, Clark's family moved to Utica, New York, where his father had taken a job with a new radio station, WRUN. That summer, while waiting to enter Syracuse University, he got his first job in radio, at WRUN, in the mimeograph and mail rooms. Before summer's end he was announcing weather forecasts, station breaks, and news. During his senior year at Syracuse University, he got a full-time announcing job at WOLF, where he disc-jockeyed country and popular music.

After graduation Clark returned to Utica, where he became the television news anchorman at WKTV. Later that year he auditioned for and won a radio

219

and TV announcing position at Philadelphia's WFIL. At WFIL Clark was soon given his own afternoon disc jockey show. In the fall of 1955 he was asked to be a substitute host on the local TV "Bandstand" show, and in 1956 he was made full-time host of that show.

In May 1957 Clark learned that the ABC Network was contemplating dropping an afternoon program of old English movies. Soon after, Ted Fetter, the network's director of programs — accompanied by Jim Aubrey, Army Grant, and Daniel Melnick, the decision-making executives at the network — visited the program in Philadelphia.

On August 5, 1957, the show made its network debut, with the new title, "American Bandstand." It has remained on the network continuously since then.

"American Bandstand" is the foundation on which Clark has built numerous other enterprises. Over the years he and his organization have been among the top producers of "live" music concerts throughout the world. They have produced as well considerable daytime and prime-time television programming, theatrical and television motion pictures, radio programming, and Dick Clark's *Good Ol' Rock 'N' Roll* revue.

Clark has also starred in three movies — *The Young Doctors, Because They Are Young,* and *Killers Three* — and has appeared in serious acting roles on dramatic shows for television. He is also the author of several books, including *Rock, Roll and Remember, Your Happiest Years, To Goof or Not to Goof, Dick Clark's Program for Success,* and *Dick Clark's The First 25 Years of Rock & Roll.*

Clark, married to the former Kari Wigton, is the father of two sons and a daughter by previous marriages. He and his wife reside in Malibu, California.

Index